D1600721

Praise for
Bioregulatory Medicine

"Sick has become the new normal as the numbers of chronically ill adults and children is ever-increasing, and patient frustration mounts as Western medicine fails to address chronic health challenges. *Bioregulatory Medicine* offers a clear and concise map on how to understand the holistic model of integrative health practice via a unified mind and body approach while supporting the individual's biology to self-regulate and regenerate. This evidence-based book takes the reader on a journey to understand how to implement a systems-focused approach to healing. This concise review is an excellent book for patients wanting to get healthy based on time-tested methods as well as for health practitioners looking to expand their own practice treatment modalities."

—**Michelle Perro**, MD,
author of *What's Making Our Children Sick?*

"I sincerely hope that the future of medicine looks much more like the approach outlined so expertly in *Bioregulatory Medicine*. Imagine a world in which each person's individuality drives the approach to treatment and good health doesn't simply mean not having any disease, but rather 'an optimized state of balance that permits a person to achieve their ultimate or highest purpose.' Luckily, this type of health care is already being practiced by doctors all over the world, and this easy-to-digest guide will open this whole world to you."

—**J.B. Handley**, author of *How to End the Autism Epidemic*

"This small book captures so many important ideas about sustainable, biologically based medicine. Its wisdom is palpable, and its science believable. To my many colleagues who, like myself, were steeped in the sciences during medical school but became disillusioned once we hit the clinical years, there is hope. This book shows us where we left our roots, which were deeply embedded in an understanding of our amazing human physiology, its intricate biochemistry, and its awe inspiring anatomy which serve as the scaffolding for each miracle of life. *Bioregulatory Medicine* is a refreshing look at what matters in medicine and how we can work *with* the human body, not against it, and without fear. We are all a complex integrated system of body-mind-spirit and, I might add, a community. Each of us is unique, each person has their own presentation and history. Thank you to all the authors who help us see what we share in common and embolden us to better care for ourselves and each other."

—**Heather Tallman Ruhm**, MD,
medical director of the Biomed Center NE

BIOREGULATORY MEDICINE

An Innovative Holistic Approach to Self-Healing

Dr. Dickson Thom, DDS, ND
Dr. James Paul Maffitt Odell, OMD, ND, L.Ac.
Dr. Jeoffrey Drobot, NMD
Dr. Frank Pleus, MD, DDS, OMFS
Jess Higgins Kelley, MNT

CHELSEA GREEN PUBLISHING
WHITE RIVER JUNCTION, VERMONT
LONDON, UK

Copyright © 2018 by Dickson Thom,
James Paul Maffitt Odell, Jeoffrey Drobot,
Frank Pleus, and Jess Higgins Kelley.
All rights reserved.

No part of this book may be transmitted or
reproduced in any form by any means without
permission in writing from the publisher.

Project Manager: Patricia Stone
Developmental Editor: Makenna Goodman
Copy Editor: Deborah Heimann
Proofreader: Laura Jorstad
Indexer: Shana Milkie
Designer: Melissa Jacobson

Printed in the United States of America.
First printing October, 2018.
10 9 8 7 6 5 4 3 2 1   18 19 20 21 22

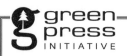

green
press
INITIATIVE

Chelsea Green Publishing is committed to preserving
ancient forests and natural resources. We elected to print
this title on 30-percent postconsumer recycled paper,
processed chlorine-free. As a result, for this printing, we
have saved:

13 Trees (40' tall and 6-8" diameter)
5.4 Million BTUs of Total Energy
5,600 Pounds of Greenhouse Gases
1,000 Gallons of Wastewater
50 Pounds of Solid Waste

Chelsea Green Publishing made this paper choice because
we and our printer, Thomson-Shore, Inc., are members
of the Green Press Initiative, a nonprofit program
dedicated to supporting authors, publishers, and suppliers
in their efforts to reduce their use of fiber obtained
from endangered forests. For more information, visit:
www.greenpressinitiative.org.

Environmental impact estimates were made using the Environmental Defense Paper Calculator.
For more information visit: www.papercalculator.org.

Our Commitment to Green Publishing

Chelsea Green sees publishing as a tool for cultural change and ecological stewardship. We strive
to align our book manufacturing practices with our editorial mission and to reduce the impact
of our business enterprise in the environment. We print our books and catalogs on chlorine-free
recycled paper, using vegetable-based inks whenever possible. This book may cost slightly more
because it was printed on paper that contains recycled fiber, and we hope you'll agree that it's
worth it. Chelsea Green is a member of the Green Press Initiative (www.greenpressinitiative.org),
a nonprofit coalition of publishers, manufacturers, and authors working to protect the world's
endangered forests and conserve natural resources. *Bioregulatory Medicine* was printed on paper
supplied by Thomson-Shore that contains at least 30% postconsumer recycled fiber.

Library of Congress Cataloging-in-Publication Data
Names: Thom, Dickson, author.
Title: Bioregulatory medicine : an innovative holistic approach to self-healing /
    Dr. Dickson Thom, DDS, ND [and four others].
Description: White River Junction, Vermont : Chelsea Green Publishing, [2018]
Identifiers: LCCN 2018028377 | ISBN 9781603588218 (paperback)
    | ISBN 9781603588225 (ebook)
Subjects: LCSH: Homeostasis. | Physiology, Pathological. | BISAC: MEDICAL / Holistic
    Medicine. | MEDICAL / Alternative Medicine. | MEDICAL / Clinical Medicine.
    | HEALTH & FITNESS / Holism.
Classification: LCC QP90.4 .T46 2018 | DDC 612/.022--dc23
LC record available at https://lccn.loc.gov/2018028377

Chelsea Green Publishing
85 North Main Street, Suite 120
White River Junction, VT 05001
(802) 295-6300
www.chelseagreen.com

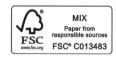

MIX
Paper from
responsible sources
FSC® C013483

CONTENTS

Patient-Focused Medicine

Today, over half of the world's population is afflicted with some form of chronic or degenerative illness—heart disease, diabetes, dementia—the list is long. Arthritis is now the most common cause of disability, and one in four people struggle with normal activities because of joint pain. Half of all people will be diagnosed with cancer in their lifetime. One in five people have an autoimmune disease. And these are just a few of the diagnosable diseases. Currently, an estimated one in ten people have a rare, undiagnosable, or medically indefinable condition. Passed like a hot potato from specialist to specialist, these tired, frustrated, and debilitated patients often spend years—not to mention significant financial resources—seeking answers, relief, and eventual cure. And the Western, conventional, allopathic, suppress-the-symptoms-with-pharmaceutical-drugs model is rapidly falling out of favor as more patients desire a nontoxic, noninvasive prevention and healing medical model that identifies and addresses the root cause of illness and elicits true healing. *Bioregulatory Medicine*, authored by five experts in the field of natural health, introduces a model that has been alive and well in Europe for decades. In countries such as Switzerland, Germany, India, China, Canada, and France—all ranking far higher in health care than the United States—*bioregulatory medicine* is a household term.

Bioregulatory medicine, or *BioMed* (both terms will be used interchangeably throughout this book), is otherwise known throughout the world as European Biological Medicine, bioregulatory systems medicine, Swiss biological medicine, or biological regulatory medicine. It is a comprehensive, evidence-based, and holistic medical model that has been used and refined for over five thousand years by some of the brightest minds in medicine, science, and philosophy. A total body (and mind) approach to health and healing, the scope of BioMed extends into disease prevention, optimizing performance, and chronic and degenerative illness treatment. Using a sophisticated synthesis of a wide range of natural and technologically advanced diagnostic and treatment equipment, BioMed aims to help facilitate and restore natural human biological processes. It is a proven, safe, gentle, highly effective, drugless, and side-effect-free medical model designed to naturally support the body to regulate, adapt, regenerate, and self-heal. What you will learn in this book is that repairing and restoring your body's systematic natural biological processes is the *only* way to prevent, reverse, and correct the deepest roots of chronic and degenerative disease. And this restoration is achieved by placing the focus on the interconnections among all the regulating systems of the body while simultaneously facilitating detoxification, deep nutrition, oral health, and nervous system calibration.

What exactly is bioregulation? For starters, the human body is comprised of approximately one hundred thousand billion cells that carry out over one hundred thousand biochemical reactions per second. Humans have dozens of bioregulating systems, including the nervous, endocrine, neurological, cardiovascular, digestive, and many more systems that we discuss in chapter 3. Every bioregulating system is intimately related on both an electrical basis and a biochemical basis to another. When communication either within or between these systems fails, dysregulation and symptoms will follow. The human body is a wondrously designed, self-regulating system that sustains all life processes, such as heart rate, blood sugar levels, hormone production, respiratory rate, detoxification, immune function, and blood pressure. Processes most of us aren't even aware are happening. Each of these systems seeks a state of balance, called homeostasis. One example of a system balancing itself is thermoregulation, where if we get too hot, we perspire. Another example is a feedback system called blood sugar regulation, where if our blood glucose gets too high, insulin is released to lower it. And if a toxin enters your system, your immune system reacts to disarm it. Breathing is regulated, blood pressure is regulated, digestion is regulated, circulation is regulated, and on and on. Consider of all the things your body is doing without you even thinking about it!

"Dis-*ease*" happens when one or more of these systems is pushed out of balance. That said, there is rarely ever a single cause of disease. Modern chronic and degenerative illnesses usually have at least five regulatory systems that are out of balance. This complexity is why there are no—and can be no—"specialists" in bioregulatory medicine: The body is interconnected. As soon as systems are viewed in isolation, we lose the whole. For example, in bioregulatory medicine, a gastroenterologist also needs to be an immunologist, because 80 percent of the immune system is located in the gastrointestinal tract. Our gut microbiota controls our mood. Hormones from the endocrine system affect the function of our digestive system. There is no cell, no system, inside our body that works independently. Because of this holistic, systems-based approach, patients new to BioMed can be surprised when immune symptoms are first approached with treatments for the brain, or skin issues are first addressed in the gastrointestinal tract. BioMed is total body medicine, which is less about treating a specific diagnosis and more about addressing and reversing dysregulation in the body as a whole.

Each bioregulatory system has an innate ability to self-repair or self-heal if injured. Think about it: A cast doesn't heal a broken arm; the biological process of bone formation called ossification does. A cast only creates one single preferred precondition—static immobilization—for a broken arm to heal. We've known about this self-healing ability for a long time. Hippocrates stated during the fifth century BC that the body has the inherent ability—the vitality—not only to heal itself and restore itself to health, but also to ward off disease. But it does this only on the condition that it's given the right tools to do so. In bioregulatory medicine, disease is not seen as the enemy with which one needs to fight, rather a manifestation of the breakdown of mechanisms that maintain control and homeostasis. Symptoms are simply the body's way of expressing dysregulation, and the goal is to identify and remove these obstacles to cure.

BioMed is about supporting and restoring the body's bioregulating systems' ability to regenerate, repair, and self-heal through the use of natural and energetic therapies. And it's even more than that, too. BioMed is a multifaceted, multidisciplinary medical model that is patient-, health-, performance-, ecology-, biology-, spiritually, physiology-, and curatively centered. Bioregulatory medicine focuses on individuality, taking into account each person's unique biochemical, historical, energetic, structural, sociological, and psycho-emotional patterns. There's only one you, so there can be only one tailored medical approach that will best meet your needs. In this way, bioregulatory medicine offers entirely customized protocols that combine ancient health care wisdom with modern scientific technological advancements. Since there is no health care manual specific to you, there is no one case study that will be similar to your process. Everyone is unique. So while allopathic medicine has strived to become an exact science, working from the platform of "hard data," just the facts, irrefutable formulas, and proven double-blind studies, bioregulatory medicine simply, artfully, and skillfully centers on the *patient*.

The diagnostics used in BioMed search beyond the conventional pathophysiological disorders of structure and function and into the arena of system regulation, as well as bioenergetic and psycho-emotional imbalances. Allopathic reliance on basic yearly blood panels and blood pressure testing just doesn't provide the type of comprehensive preventive screening required to properly assess complex chronic and degenerative illness. The diagnostics of bioregulatory medicine are unsurpassed, using innovations from heart rate variability testing, comprehensive hormone and digestion function testing, contact regulation thermography (CRT), digital pulsewave analysis (DPA), electrodermal testing, food allergy and sensitivity testing, and beyond. In one visit with a BioMed doctor, a patient might get a centuries-old diagnostic approach, such as Chinese medicine tongue analysis, and also the modern German technological innovations found in bioresonance testing. Both are highly effective, noninvasive, and nontoxic methods of detecting early signs of degenerative disease within an organ, systemic inflammation, or various infections. These, and all other diagnostic tools used in BioMed (alongside standard blood chemistry testing), can detect early signs of disease. One highly attractive element of the bioregulatory medical model is its noninvasive prevention capabilities: Testing is fast, painless, and nontoxic. Testing detects disease patterns before they start, and catches them before they progress.

Beyond being the premier prevention-focused medical model for adults, bioregulatory medical testing is also the go-to for pediatric patients who generally aren't too keen about getting poked and prodded, but are sadly becoming more and more afflicted by an epidemic of chronic disease.

Once patients are tested, and if disease or dysregulation patterns are present, the paradigm of bioregulatory medicine treatment is centered on changing the patient's bioregulatory terrain, also known as the internal milieu. The state of our bioindividual internal and external ecosystems spells the difference between health and disease. BioMed treatments aim to optimize the state of the patient's terrain, facilitating healing as safely and effectively as possible in order to restore homeostasis in all the body's bioregulatory systems. When the terrain is healthy, it becomes an inhospitable place for dysregulation and disease to take hold. This positions terrain-focused bioregulatory medicine as the most elite, comprehensive medical model when it comes to prevention, optimal performance, personalized medicine, and the treatment of chronic and degenerative illness. As Dr. Samuel Hahnemann, the father of homeopathic medicine, said: "The highest ideal of cure is rapid, gentle and permanent restoration of health, and removal or annihilation of the disease in its whole extent in the shortest, most reliable, and most harmless way, on easily comprehensible principles."[1]

BioMed is about support and stimulation—working with biology through biological means. Thus, one of the primary premises of bioregulatory medicine is the doctrine of *vis medicatrix naturae*, or "the healing power of nature," which refers to the inherent self-organizing and self-healing processes of all living organisms. With

BioMed, the more nontoxic the treatments to help accomplish the healing and cure, the better. (Interestingly, the term *physician* has Latin roots and means "things relating to nature." How far away that definition feels when speaking to a synthetic-pharmaceutical-prescribing allopathic physician!) Bioregulatory medicine is about treating living humans with biological, synergetic, symbiotic, and organic medicines that our bodies and genetics have evolved with for hundreds of thousands of years.

Even Western allopathic medicine has tried jumping on the bioregulatory medicine bandwagon in their own way. Allopathic medicine has adopted (confusingly) the term *biologic drugs* to describe a new class of pharmaceuticals, most of which are genetically engineered viruses and antibodies derived from human, animal, or microbial origins. Allopathic practitioners realized patients understand the need to attend to biological wisdom and so the system co-opted the terminology. Their hope is no one will notice. Sadly the majority of these patented biologic drugs act *opposite* to the bioregulatory medicine foundational concept of "maintenance and furtherance of the human biosystem and its regulatory mechanisms." Biologic drugs, more appropriately termed *biopharmaceuticals*, have been altered from their natural state in order to be patented and marketable, yet have been rendered unlike biological molecules found in nature. Therefore, they do not act in the body the way natural plant-based and energetic medicines and treatments do. But because biologically sourced medicines are both powerful and profitable to the pharmaceutical industry, they continue to be researched, manufactured, and marketed under the nomenclature of so-called biologic drugs. As of 2016, biopharmaceuticals surged to make up 25 percent of the total pharmaceutical market, raking in $232 billion. Their name makes them sound like they are natural and harmless, but they are not. Therefore it is important that bioregulatory medicine and its natural biological remedies and therapies not be confused with the pharmacological agents conventional medicine now calls "biologic drugs."

True bioregulatory medicine uses naturally occurring and energetically active compounds that have the safest and greatest biological effect on humans. They work in harmony with the body as opposed to against it. Keeping pace with constant technological advancements, bioregulatory medicine incorporates the best of the natural, classical, time-tested treatment modalities and the modern and high-tech technological treatment modalities the world has to offer, including Chinese medicine; anthroposophical medicine; antihomotoxic therapy; homeopathy; bioenergetic therapy; electromagnetic field therapy; phytotherapy; hyperthermia; organotherapy; oxygen therapy; ozone therapy; sound, light, and energy therapies; genetic, metabolic, psychosomatic, dental, nutritional, and herbal treatments; as well as various structural, postural, and bioenergetic therapies. Most importantly, every single treatment is aimed to support an individual's ability to regulate, adapt, regenerate, and self-heal. Where many patients find themselves frustrated and hopping from one natural medicine practitioner to the next, the strength of the BioMed clinics in the United States is that they offer *all* of these diagnostics and treatments—many of which you can't access anywhere outside of Europe—under one roof. This is an exciting moment for BioMed. Finally, patients no longer need to travel to Europe to access state-of-the-art, innovative, nontoxic, and noninvasive treatments. So laypeople fed up with being fed piles of pharmaceuticals, including high-ranking CEOs, hedge fund managers, and professional athletes, are flocking to these clinics.

For the sake of comparison to an already established model in the United States, bioregulatory medicine is most closely related to vitalistic naturopathic medicine. The vitalism theory states that organic, biological materials contain the "vital force" of life and are therefore the best-suited type of medicine to support human biology. Biological (*bios* means "life") medicine cures humans, or biological beings. In contrast, synthetic, xenotoxic, or nonnatural materials—including most pharmaceuticals—are foreign to the body, and therefore will not have the vital force to elicit a healing or curative response. (More on this in chapter 4.) Meanwhile, many naturopathic physicians in the United States are already practicing bioregulatory medicine, and either they don't know it or they just haven't been able to place where the connections they've been making in their own practices have been offered as an American medical discipline.

It is also important to note that "integrative medicine" is a new movement started only in the last twenty years or so, by naturopathic or otherwise alternative doctors that want to play nice with the allopathic world and integrate pharmaceutical medicine alongside natural medicine. While this is an important step in the right direction, the harm caused by many pharmaceutical drugs on a mitochondrial level goes against bioregulatory medicine's continued embodiment of the Hippocratic Oath sworn by all physicians (at least, historically) of *Do No Harm*. Bioregulatory medicine is on the leading edge of natural medicine, honoring the vital force in us while also applying the power of modern testing and technology alongside classical healing traditions. The use of highly toxic and synthetic practices, even when in combination with alternative therapies, ultimately undermines our health. The more gentle and noninvasive the therapy, the less disruptive it will be to the patient's integral whole.

In fact, many BioMed treatments are so subtle, people have a hard time believing they actually work. When we introduce many of the bioregulatory treatment methods and machines to new patients, they often seem exotic or implausible, our allopathically programmed minds just can't believe they work. The use of energy, frequency, and light are just a few of the modalities that bioregulatory medicine uses to stimulate self-healing, and sometimes these are too abstract for newcomers to fully grasp. It's similar to trying to understand quantum physics without a background in science—complex. This book aims to teach you the basics of how this works. It's time to open our minds to modern and advanced approaches to treatment that push the edge of bioregulatory medicine.

Bioregulatory medicine's introduction to the United States is well timed, as we are currently seeing a clear division in naturopathic practice in the United States. It might surprise readers to know that today many naturopathic schools are phasing out education in holistic treatments in order to teach allopathic pharmacology and pathology. The result is this: Even natural doctors are being educated to view health and disease through an allopathic lense. It is important to know that the term *allopathy* means "the treatment of disease by remedies that produce effects *opposite* to the symptoms." Allopathic treatments are intended to replace, remove, destroy, block, suppress, or inhibit biological function, not to support the body's natural healing process. Allopathic medicine is not natural medicine.

For example, consider Patient #1, who has a low-functioning thyroid as determined by a TSH test alone: She walks into her allopathic doctor's office and is prescribed Synthroid, a synthetic thyroid hormone replacement drug. Patient #2, with the same issue, walks into her naturopath's office and gets Nature-Throid, a natural thyroid hormone replacement drug. Patient #3 has the same issue and walks into her integrative physician's office and gets one or the other of the same drugs (natural or synthetic) and maybe some zinc. But Patient #4 walks into her bioregulatory physician's office and gets a complete thyroid panel with antibody testing, heavy-metal testing, complete hormone analysis, and nervous system testing and is prescribed a corrective diet; supplemental vitamins, minerals and glandulars; energy treatments including acupuncture; and more, depending on her unique history and biochemical makeup. Nature-Throid, while *seemingly* more natural, is no different than the conventional Synthroid—it is a drug that does not seek to cure the underlying thyroid imbalance, but rather seeks to mask the symptoms with a one-target, one-drug approach. The solution is not as simple as just replacing the "bad" with the "good."

A bioregulatory medicine physician takes into account a person's history even from before birth. The elements and experiences that make up a patient's unique emotional, physical, and spiritual life tapestry all must be accounted for. Is the thyroid dysfunction a result of exposure to heavy metals or is it from overexposure to dry cleaning agents? Is it from a gluten intolerance or from an autoimmune process? Is it due to childhood trauma, or to a lack of finding one's "voice"? Sometimes, it's all of these. This complexity is why bioregulatory medicine utilizes a multidiagnostic approach in order to discover *all* the causative factors involved in an illness in order to best formulate a customized individualized treatment plan.

Here's another example: Two women who are the same age and share the same breast cancer diagnosis will get the same toxic treatment protocol in allopathic medicine. Yet their unique biochemical, emotional, and physical processes that led to the disease were likely very different, regardless of the seemingly similar diagnosis. Perhaps one woman had chronic exposure to highly toxic building materials and experienced depression while the other was overweight, diabetic, and suffered chronic constipation. In a bioregulatory medicine practice, each of these women would receive different nontoxic treatments tailored entirely to their individual terrain. While patients might have the same disease or prognosis, the manifestation of illness is entirely bioindividual and must be treated and prevented on a personalized level. That said, all of the treatments listed in this book are used in many, many different combinations and integrations determined specifically to the individual. This is personalized medicine.

Bioregulatory medicine therapeutics and treatments are designed to cure and heal, not replace, suppress, block, or inhibit. So next time your doctor recommends a medication, ask if it will heal the condition itself or if it will just suppress the symptoms. This is also a question for a supplement-focused naturopathic physician: Is Nature-Throid curing the thyroid condition, or is it just a more natural version of a synthetic palliative drug? Even in natural and integrative medicine models, if a physician sees a patient's symptom improving with supplement use, the patient is directed to "keep doing what she is doing," and then is confined to taking a supplement or pharmaceutical for the rest of their life. But taking a pile of supplements every day does not stop whatever multiple factors are driving the imbalance, is not a well-defined cure, and can lead to further complications in the future. Reevaluation and retesting of a patient's individual situation and readapting the treatment plan is a must in BioMed. Good medicine is about getting to the cause, whatever might be blocking or causing imbalances to bioregulation, and removing it—whether it is toxic overload, poor nutrition, an imbalanced nervous system, or oral infections.

If you were to think of disease as a stone in your sandal, allopathic medicine would prescribe a synthetic pharmaceutical that would eliminate the pain, allowing you to walk, while bioregulatory medicine would remove the stone. Simplicity is an important but often overlooked element in the art of effective medicine. Yet allopathic medicine is glued to a reductionist and mechanically minded thought process that views the body as parts separated from the whole. The neurologist and the gastroenterologist might send you to the cardiologist or the endocrinologist, but likely none of them are talking to each other. This is a problem, because all the systems in your body *do* talk to each other, and it is our job to listen. When it comes to the profundity of chronic and degenerative illness, medical specialization is like blind men looking at an elephant—one thinks it's a wall, the other a tree. With the 20/20 vision offered by holistic medicine, a bioregulatory physician incorporates all medical specialties into one treatment plan *and* offers a complete understanding of the interactions among these systems.

This book is meant for forward-thinking practitioners and patients looking for a modern natural approach to health care. It is meant as a general introduction to bioregulatory medicine, so readers should consider it a jumping-off point for further research, experimentation, or education at one of the Bioregulatory Medicine Institute's clinics. In the first two chapters we question the efficacy and safety of the pharmaceutical-based allopathic medical approach while contrasting it with the age-old safety record of BioMed. Despite how new allopathic medicine is in the context of the history of medicine, its financial prowess has shoved all other natural medical sects to the sidelines—labeling them as "alternative." Actually, BioMed has roots in the oldest forms of evidence-based medicine. Throughout the first few chapters you will gain a clear sense of how different allopathy and bioregulatory are in both prevention and treatment approaches: Bioregulatory medicine works with the body, allopathy works against the body. Consider the flu. In allopathic medicine, the flu is prevented with toxic vaccinations and treated with anti-inflammatories and antivirals that suppress or block biological processes. Bioregulatory medicine prevents the flu by fortifying the terrain with immune-boosting nutrients and herbs, proper rest, and stress-reduction techniques and treats the flu with acupuncture, warming herbs, hydrotherapy, garlic, and medicinal broths. This book will help answer the question: Which of these sounds better to you?

In chapter 3 we detail the foundational concepts behind bioregulatory medicine's unified systems-based approach to self-healing. Bioregulatory medicine restores the body's dozen bioregulating systems' ability to respond, react, and adapt to the daily stressors of everyday life and return to balance, or homeostasis. In chapters 4 through 7 we dive into the four primary therapeutic pillars of bioregulatory medicine: detox and drainage, nutrition, nervous system calibration, and oral health. In chapter 8 you will find an introductory list and brief descriptions of the many ancient and newer diagnostics and treatments used by bioregulatory medicine

We encourage you to open your mind, as many of these modalities might seem foreign or might even have been disregarded by your allopathic physician. Sadly, we've been ingrained, bought, and taught by the pharmaceutical, chemical, and allopathic marketing models that drugs, radiation, and surgery are the only valid medical treatments. Anything else is labeled unorthodox or dangerous, has no validity, or is "unconventional." This mindset is gravely incorrect and is propelled by the fear-based model of conventional allopathy—fear of unvaccination, fear of our genes, fear of germs, fear of disease, fear of the flu. This mindset is a cover-up: A 2018 Johns Hopkins study concluded that medical errors are the third-leading cause of death after heart disease and cancer.[2] What sounds scarier to you? A natural, nontoxic medicine used successfully for thousands of years or a synthetic poison used for thirty years that hasn't been properly tested? Get ready for a whole new view and approach to health and healing.

CHAPTER ONE

Modern Disease and the Rise of the Allopathic Model

Every body continues in its state of rest, or of uniform motion in a right line, unless it is compelled to change that state by forces impressed upon it.

—SIR ISAAC NEWTON

The art of medicine consists of amusing the patient while nature cures the disease.

—VOLTAIRE

C hronic and degenerative illnesses are largely new to mankind. In fact, diseases such as cancer, diabetes, fibromyalgia, and multiple sclerosis have been termed *modern* or *man-made* diseases because they were relatively rare until three hundred years or so ago. The term *chronic illness* (versus *acute illness*, such as the bubonic plague or a broken arm) comes from the Greek god of time, Chronos, and can be defined as an illness that persists for a long time, usually more than three months, and is often slow in its progression. The environment for these illnesses can be set early; many chronic diseases have traceable roots in childhood. Cancer, for example, can take decades of development before becoming a diagnosable mass. Chronic illnesses, such as Alzheimer's disease, start with a degenerative process—a gradual deterioration of specific tissues, cells, or organs. This causes loss of function or structure—for the mind in Alzheimer's, the bones in osteoporosis. Little by little things get worse.

In disease, cells degenerate, meaning they no longer generate sufficient energy for proper functioning and health. Put simply, the body runs out of battery power, or out of gas. The switch might be flipped on, but there's no light to be seen. In the body, the cellular batteries that provide operating power are molecules called adenosine triphosphate, or ATP, sometimes referred to as the energy currency of life. ATP is created in the mitochondria, which are tiny yet oh-so-powerful energy-producing factories within the nucleus of each cell. Here's what is important about mitochondria: Cutting-edge medical research has found that chronic and degenerative diseases share *one* thing in common: dysregulated energy production.[1] In other words, the mitochondria have stopped functioning as they should, like an engine without an alternator. In fact, the numerous conditions that involve mitochondrial dysfunction include: diabetes, Huntington's disease, cancer, Alzheimer's disease, Parkinson's disease, bipolar disorder, schizophrenia, aging, anxiety disorders, cardiovascular disease, and chronic fatigue syndrome.[2] Energy—or the lack thereof—is the difference between health and disease, life and death. This fact is why the central focus of BioMed is on the use of biologically energetic (alive) diagnostics and therapeutics.

The modern diseases we face are multifactorial, meaning they are caused by many contributing factors with dysregulation and degeneration at their roots. Dysregulation is caused when our bioregulating systems are pushed away or blocked from the normal state of balance, or homeostasis. Common symptoms of bioregulatory dysregulation can include allergies, inflammation, pain, headaches, exhaustion, depression, tension, sleeplessness, indigestion, and recurrent infections. These classic symptoms are often a response to an overload of prescription drugs, toxic chemicals, pollution, poor-quality or allergenic foods, psycho-emotional stress, lack of exercise, nutrient deficiencies, and dental infections—all of which can damage the mitochondria when they persist over time. Pharmaceutical medications are now also known as a major contributor to mitochondrial damage, which explains all the adverse (also known as "side") effects. In fact, all classes of psychotropic drugs, as well as statin medications and analgesics such as acetaminophen, have been documented to damage mitochondria.[3] Considering that many people with chronic illness have been on these drugs for years, and sometimes for decades, we're talking about a high level of mitochondrial damage.

The allopathic medical model's staunch dogmatic entrenchment in the one-size-fits-all drugs-for-everyone paradigm isn't getting to the energetic roots of modern diseases. This model implies that if you take a Tylenol for a headache and the pain goes away, you can assume the headache was due to a Tylenol deficiency. Yet estimates show that 85 percent of chronic and degenerative diseases are rooted in adaptable elements such as diet, lifestyle, mitochondrial function, and emotional well-being. And this model is exactly why we are losing the war on cancer, why multiple sclerosis patients slowly but surely lose significant function, and why chronic fatigue syndrome has become the biggest blanket diagnosis of our time. Headache? Take a Tylenol. Backache? Have some oxycodone. Prevention is not the focus and palliation is not a cure, because when you stop taking the drug, the symptoms return. The immediate-gratification, take-two-aspirin-and-call-me-in-the-morning allopathic approach doesn't cure chronic or degenerative illnesses. We deserve better medicine than this.

Yet without even realizing it, we've become entrenched in allopathy. Since the widespread adoption of the current health care model in the 1960s (when HMO and private insurance were introduced during the time of President Nixon), medical costs have escalated as much as fifteen-fold, while rates of chronic disease are projected to increase more than 50 percent by 2023. We've spent significant amounts of money, but not much progress has been made. The US health care system is ranked the worst among the eleven developed nations. Meanwhile, Canada, Denmark, Sweden, Switzerland, and Germany top the charts. What are they doing differently? Many things, of course, but the commonality between these other countries is the use of bioregulatory medicine practices. In the United States it's time for a more comprehensive and sophisticated medical model, one especially adapted to the current complexities of chronic illnesses. The "just wait until it's broken," with little regard to prevention or sharpening health, is a sick-care model that no longer satisfies most US citizens. But do we even know what true health is anymore?

What Is Health, Anyway?

The allopathic definition of health sets the bar pretty low. *Health is generally defined as a physical and mental state free from illness, disease, or symptoms.* Does that seem good enough to you? Are we supposed to think that anything other than sick is "healthy"? Should we wait until we are diagnosed with a disease before we pay attention to our health? Yet this low-bar definition is exactly why when people do get a diagnosis, the most common phrase uttered is *But I was so healthy before I got diagnosed!* Really, most of us are not at our peak health, even when we think we are. The problem is our annual physical exams aren't looking to optimize health; they are merely screening for disease. The allopathic approach to disease prevention and early detection is elementary at best. Reviewing basic lab reports, checking blood pressure, heart rate, and temperature are part of a static, in-the-moment assessment of our body's complex and historical picture. In the allopathic model, if a lab marker is outside the "reference range," it is enough to justify a diagnosis, which today means also receiving a pharmaceutical prescription.

Of course, there's no money in preventing disease. US drug sales are projected to reach $610 billion by 2021.[4] It is no stretch of the imagination to say that true and lasting health promises little financial gain. When allopathic medicine does embrace prevention, it's usually in the form of profitable pharmaceuticals or screenings: baby aspirin to prevent cardiovascular disease, statins to prevent high cholesterol, annual flu shots, the list goes on. Radiation-based screenings such as mammograms, which can confer false positives and have even been shown to be a *cause* of breast cancer, are generally the only breast cancer prevention option presented to women.[5] But this is not prevention, it's almost a *preparation* for the disease. Pills, vaccinations, and screenings are only aimed at finding a diagnosable condition that will convert into profit-making conventional treatments such as drugs, surgery, or radiation. The allopathic focus of health is truly on disease. It is a disease-centric model.

In direct contrast, bioregulatory medicine views health as much more than merely the *absence* of symptoms or disease. Instead, in BioMed, *health* is defined as a state of "complete physical, mental, and social well-being." *Well-being* is defined as a "mode of being comfortable, balanced, mindful, healthy, and happy." Health is an optimized state of balance that permits a person to achieve their ultimate or highest purpose. It's not about feeling *just okay*, it's about feeling *your best*. Bioregulatory medicine is a model centered on both health and prevention, taking into full account a phrase from the Hippocratic Oath: *I will prevent disease whenever I can, for prevention is preferable to cure.* The diagnostics and screenings used in bioregulatory medicine draw upon nontoxic technologies that also take into account the cross talk between bioregulating systems. For example, a heart rate variability monitor and assessment device can determine how stress (which we all have) is affecting both the heart and the nervous system, and this data can predict potential future health problems. This test takes about five minutes and is completely noninvasive.

The Suppression-Addiction Prescription

Western allopathic medicine relies on drugs that result in an *opposite* effect of the symptoms. From Greek roots, *allopathic* literally means "opposite of disease." The model is based on using drugs that work *against* our biology to suppress disease symptoms. Here lies the fundamental distinction: Allopathic medicine treatments suppress biology while bioregulatory medicine supports it. BioMed is the embodiment of symbiotic medicine, whereas allopathic medicine is antagonistic medicine. Waves of "prove-it" research are beginning to confirm what bioregulatory medicine's roots have always known: that the body's natural ability to heal is profound and should be facilitated, not suppressed. To be clear, there is no question that allopathic medicine in the United States offers some of the finest acute care globally. It has succeeded in reducing the ravages of infectious disease and developed incredibly innovative surgical procedures and synthetic drugs. If you shatter your arm or get an acute infection, an American hospital is where you want to be. But when it comes to chronic and degenerative illnesses, the American conventional medical model is stuck in suppression as the standard of care.

Suppression of symptoms curtails a normal flow, discharge, action, or interaction by removing, blocking, or inhibiting a normal biological action. Antihistamines block watery eyes and stuffy nose. Statin drugs inhibit the enzyme HMG-CoA reductase, which plays a central role in the production of cholesterol. While these therapies do indeed stop the patient's symptoms, the suppression only results in the creation of a deeper dysfunction. If you keep shoving dirt under the carpet for long enough, eventually you have a huge mess. For example, a 2010 study in the *American Journal of Respiratory and Critical Care Medicine* found that suppressing fevers with Tylenol is responsible for as many as four in ten cases of wheezing and severe asthma in teens.[6] BioMed recognizes the healing power of a fever (to a safe extent), and even harnesses heat in treatments such as hyperthermia. Long-term use of antihistamines has been found to cause dementia.[7] Yet we know that increased seasonal allergies (why people look to antihistamines in the first place) are a direct result of toxic diets and nutritional deficiencies that BioMed looks to restore. Long-term statin use—ten years or longer—more than doubles women's risk of invasive ductal carcinoma and invasive lobular carcinoma.[8] Many users of medication for high blood pressure and statin drugs have heart attacks, suggesting that the medications are not helpful and, in fact, from a biological processes viewpoint, are doing more harm than good. The sad truth is that the standard of care in the United States is a symptom-suppressing, disease-focused model with little nod to true underlying causes or long-term healing.

Many of the drugs prescribed today were discovered and developed within the past one hundred years, which is a tiny speck of time in the life cycle of medicine. The era of cancer chemotherapy, for example, began in the early 1900s, after World War I, when chemicals became king. By happenstance it was observed that a toxic agent of war called mustard gas could also inhibit cell division and growth. So the American medical establishment said: *Let's try it on cancer cells!* Today a derivative of mustard gas, thiotepa, is used as a cancer-treatment drug, but it is also classified as a Group 1 human carcinogen by the World Health Organization. How can something be considered a medicine and a disease-causing agent at the same time? We can do better than fighting disease with agents known to cause disease, especially considering estimates show the majority of all chronic illness cases are caused by diet, lifestyle, or unfavorable environmental cofactors.[9] It's time patients had more treatment options than toxic pharmaceutical drugs and invasive procedures. Of course, chemotherapy does push back cancer in *some* cases. But those who survive it are often left with long-term side effects such as brain fog or neuropathy. Is this the only way? While the undesirable effects that come from synthetic pharmaceutical drug use are called *side effects*, they should really be termed *adverse* effects, and in some cases, *addictive* effects.

Currently, the most commonly prescribed—and abused— medications of our time are opioids. Called the joy plant, extracts from the delicate pink-leaved opium poppy act on opioid receptors to produce pain-relieving effects. Cultivation of the poppy plant has been happening since 3400 BC. Today there are approximately ten classes of poppy-derivative drugs approved for use in the management of pain in the United States and Canada. And then there is the illegal version: heroin. The misuse of and addiction to opioids has become a very serious national crisis. With fentanyl, hydrocodone, morphine, oxycodone, and heroin all in use, each day more than ninety Americans die from opioid overdose. Much of this opioid addiction and overdose is a direct result of overprescription. In the United States there were 240 million opioid prescriptions dispensed in 2015, nearly one for every adult in the general population.[10] The opioid situation in America is a classic example of a health crisis *caused* by allopathic medical care.

Yet the biggest snag in medicine is that since a plant cannot technically be patented, the drug industry is highly incentivized to "invent" synthetic drugs. Ironically, many of these aim to achieve the efficacy of, and are sometimes derived from, biologically active plants.

Poppy plant to oxycodone is a perfect example. In fact, up to 50 percent of the FDA-approved drugs during the last forty years were derived either directly or indirectly from natural products.[11] However, this does not mean pharmaceuticals are inherently "natural." From plant to pill most pharmaceuticals are synthetic (read: foreign to our bodies), so they can and do cause adverse effects. Today, nearly three in five American adults take prescription drugs—one often to offset the effects of another. If a drug is the "cure," then allopathic medicine tells us that to be cured really means to be medicated.

Consider corticosteroids such as hydrocortisone, prednisolone, and cortisol. These medications were invented in the 1930s, almost one hundred years ago, and they remain some of the most widely prescribed drugs for their many opposing effects: anti-inflammatory, immunosuppressive, antiproliferative, and vasoconstrictive. Steroids decrease inflammation, and so are largely prescribed for rheumatoid arthritis and many other conditions. They also reduce the activity of the immune system and so are widely used in allopathic medicine for autoimmune conditions. And while steroid prescriptions are written hand over fist, the medical doctors prescribing them make money. In the United States about 75 percent of medical doctors received at least one payment from a drug or equipment company in 2014, according to a ProPublica analysis. That same year, Americans were handed 4.3 billion prescriptions.[12] Palliation is the prescription for profit.

That leaves us here: When it comes to the allopathic medical treatment for chronic and degenerative diseases, we should be asking ourselves this question: Is it healing or hurting? Estimates suggest that allopathic medicine is responsible for 128,000 deaths per year in the United States; almost half of those are from adverse reactions to prescription drugs (predominantly opioids), and more than 250,000 deaths per year are due to medical error.[13] In fact, the most common reason Americans go to the doctor is to deal with their medications. This is health? There is a pill for everything, and pharmaceutical drugs are often the only treatment option offered. Sure, from a psychological standpoint, this pop-a-pill-and-get-on-with-it approach *is* the right match for our fast-paced society. Most

Americans "don't have time" to wait for a cure. A quick fix is good enough for now! And why not? Access to almost anything can be fast: food, information, sex, drugs. Why wait for health when a pill can stop it now? Certainly there is no question that providing relief from uncomfortable and debilitating symptoms is an important element of medicine. But there are better ways to alleviate pain than to overmedicate. Bioregulatory medicine, like allopathic medicine, utilizes many different modalities to reduce symptoms, but only to buy time while other restorative and regenerative treatments activate, restore, and repair the body's intrinsic healing mechanisms. While drugs help palliate, the body also needs to be energetically stimulated to detoxify, regulate, balance, regenerate, replenish, and finally heal, and this is exactly what bioregulatory medicine does. Yet true healing is no quick fix; it can take months or years to rebuild and regenerate. So why has this kind of deeply rooted medicine been unavailable in the United States for so long? To answer this important question, we need a historical platform by which to view the evolution of various medical sects, approaches, and philosophies.

Origins of Medical Theories, Philosophies, and Sects

The world's oldest medical systems are India's Ayurveda and China's traditional Chinese medicine (TCM), both dating back almost six thousand years. The focus of both these models—and from where BioMed pulls its oldest roots—is on the *patient* rather than the disease. Promoting health and enhancing the quality of life in each of these medical systems has been accomplished through the use of therapeutic strategies applied in a holistic fashion. Holistic medicine views the body as a complete internal and external system that reacts to its environment. These ancient healing models focus also on the mind, spirit, and emotions. Holistic medicine is far from a new concept; it's the oldest medical model there is.

Both Ayurveda and TCM also view health and disease in relation to energy. *Prana*, referred to in Ayurveda, means "life energy," and *qi* (pronounced "chi"), from TCM, means the body's "vital force."

Energy has been an integral part of health since the beginning of medicine; today we call it mitochondria or biofields. Throughout this book you will learn that energy is the not-so-secret key to health. In fact, the energy-is-medicine torch was lit in antediluvian China and India then migrated west to Greece, where its recognition continued to burn.

Around six thousand years ago medicine emerged from caves of the occult and crept into the temples of philosophy. Hippocrates of Kos, considered the father of modern medicine, proposed that medicine was largely influenced by the human connection to nature and *pneuma*, the Greek term for energy or natural force. Hippocrates developed a medical theory (one that pervaded societies for thousands of years) that nature's four elements—water, earth, wind, and fire—had an analogous relationship to the body. These elements were reflected in the body by four fluids called humors: black bile, yellow bile, phlegm, and blood. Pneuma is infused into each of these four humors, powering their respective functions and actions. Symptoms and disease thus arose when there was an excess—or a lack—of one of these humors. Hippocrates defined the duty of the physician as to reinstate a balance of these humors by helping facilitate the healing virtues of nature and our body's innate ability to heal.

The first to attest to the Law of Similars, Hippocrates asserted that using treatments that encouraged the same symptoms would encourage healing. He said, "By similar things a disease is produced and through the application of the like is cured." Conditions such as fevers, in other words, should be treated with heat. The common cold can be treated with various applications of cold water. Hippocrates demonstrated that disease, in fact, is a natural process, and that symptoms are natural reactions of the body to a disease process. He recognized the mind-body connection and advocated therapies including a healthy diet, a balanced lifestyle, and botanical medicines. His famous quote "Let food be thy medicine and medicine be thy food" is still widely used in nutritional medicine today, and was a part of the original Hippocratic Oath. But of course, questioning is the hallmark of philosophy, and eventually the Law of Similars was challenged.

Claudius Galen, a Greek physician, surgeon, and philosopher in the Roman Empire, also largely steered the course of medicine, but in a different philosophic direction. Like Hippocrates, he believed in the healing power of nature, but in stark contrast, Galen introduced the idea of treatment by opposites, known as the Law of Contraries. If a patient appeared with a fever, they were treated with something cold. This doctrine provided the foundation of allopathic medicine. From the Greek word *allos*, or "other," allopathic medicine is the method of treating a disease with a remedy that produces effects differing from those produced by the disease itself. With Galen we saw the first division of medical philosophy: one school of thought working in accordance with biology, the other working in its opposition. Just like in American politics, proponents of each of these sides have been debating each other for thousands of years. And just as medical philosophy has undergone profound question and evolution, so has medicine itself.

The Apothecary, the Pharmacy, and Homeopathy

Pharmacology is the branch of medicine that studies the uses, effects, and actions of drugs. It is a term derived from the Greek word *pharmakon*, meaning "poison" in classic Greek and "drug" in modern Greek. The essence of pharmacology is to examine the interaction between a living organism and a specific compound, and observe any normal or abnormal biochemical or metabolic activities. From cauldron to Coke bottle this field of study is as old as mankind. The earliest known documentation of pharmacological substances is the *Sushruta Samhita*, an Indian Ayurvedic treatise from the sixth century BC that describes hundreds of medicinal herbs, including their safety, efficacy, dosage, and benefits. From ancient Egypt, the *Ebers Papyrus*, dating back to the third century BC, lists the extensive plant- and animal-derived pharmacopeia used by that civilization, including myrrh, juniper berries, poppy, lead, salt, lizard's blood, embalming essential oils, and various excreta. Medicine, since the beginning of time, has been derived from biological, natural substances that were studied for their pharmacological action.

Around AD 60, Pedanius Dioscorides, a first-century Greek physician, botanist, and pharmacologist, wrote *De Materia Medica*, which became the foremost source of modern botanical terminology and the leading pharmacological text for the next sixteen centuries. Crowned the father of pharmacology, Dioscorides was first a military physician whose hobby was to study medicinal plants wherever he traveled. His five-volume encyclopedia described how to prepare medicine from various plant parts and when each part should be harvested for maximum efficacy. Plants included pine bark, pepper, opium, belladonna, poppy, buttercup, jimsonweed, henbane, and deadly nightshade.[14] For all of human history, until the last few hundred years, plants, animals, and minerals were the foundation for all druglike substances—working both with and against biology depending on the medical sect with which the physician was aligned.

During the Middle Ages in Europe knowledge and interest in medicinal plants grew. Botanical gardens began to sprout, and pharmacylike shops that formulated and dispensed *materia medica*, which were called apothecaries, also cropped up. Interest in medicine was increasing as disease was becoming more virulent. The Black Death, one of the most devastating pandemics in human history, killed almost 60 percent of Europe's population between 1346 and 1353. By that time, medicine had settled quite comfortably into the theories of the four humors and the Law of Contraries. So when Paracelsus came on the scene in the fifteenth century, he gave Hippocratic medicine a much-needed revival and provocative stir.

A Swiss physician, alchemist, and astrologer of the German Renaissance, Paracelsus (born Theophrastus von Hohenheim) called for a return to the Hippocratic view of "like cures like." So adamant was Paracelsus that he burned the books of Galen, causing rampant feather flapping in a world nested in an allopathic focus. Paracelsus further aimed to resurrect the nature cure focus of the early Greeks. He argued that while the body was a chemical system that had to be balanced internally, it also needed to be in harmony with its environment. Paracelsus not only proposed a chemistry and energetic approach to cure, but also introduced a new class of *materia medica*, including metallic and mineral substances. He was noted for saying, "Poison is in everything, and no thing is without poison. The dosage makes it either a poison or a remedy." Using this dosage mindset, he first introduced the concept of using potentially toxic remedies to elicit a cure. Mercury, lead, arsenic, and antimony—poisons to most—were cures in his view. His use of these substances to cure diseases of the times crowned him as the father of toxicology.

On the historical heels of Paracelcus, Samuel Hahnemann, a German physician born in 1755, furthered the like-cures-like legacy spawned by Hippocrates. Hahnemann believed in the detailed testing of drugs on healthy human bodies to obtain valid knowledge of a drug's effects. He went as far as to self-experiment with the antimalarial drug quinine, derived from the bark of the cinchona tree. He discovered that the drug had a similar effect to the illness it was supposed to cure—in a healthy person, a dose of quinine caused a fever. Hahnemann developed the central idea of homeopathic medicine (from the Greek word, *homoios*, meaning "like" or "resembling"). Homeopathic medicine is based on the age-old principle that the body is able to heal itself, and that like cures like. The first homeopathic hospital opened in 1832 in Leipzig, Germany, followed by several others throughout Europe. While serving on the faculty at Leipzig University, Hahnemann became disillusioned with the emerging standard medical practices of the time, including overdrugging and bloodletting. He pursued instead the "natural laws" of medicine, opposing allopathy, and further developed the Law of Similars (*similia similibus curantur*). During the mid-1800s, the foundations of Hippocratic and bioregulatory medicine were confirmed and practiced. That is, until science shoved medicine under a microscope, disease became microbial, and the lights in Hippocratic medical schools were turned off.

It Must Be Proven to Be True:
The Rise of Empiricism

Empiricism, or the theory that knowledge only comes from what we can confirm with our senses, appealed to the plague-stricken populations of the fifteenth through eighteenth centuries. It became a fundamental part of the prevailing scientific method, dictating that all hypotheses and theories must be tested against observations of the natural world rather than on reasoning, intuition, revelation, or anecdotal evidence. Empiricism states that methods must be *proven* to be true, regardless of the anecdotal evidence used for thousands of years. So, for example, where physicians had always confirmed the importance of the spiritual aspect of medicine, philosophers such as René Descartes heralded in the concept of mind-body dualism instead: that the mind and body are two distinct entities. Medicine, therefore, according to Descartes should focus only on the physical body, because, unlike the mind, the body is observable and objectified. The mind and spirit should be ignored because they cannot be quantified. Descartes, aptly dubbed the father of modern Western philosophy, believed that an idea with any doubt should be rejected entirely, and accepted only if it acquired a firm foundation of knowledge and validity. English philosopher Francis Bacon, an ally in this view, declared that the aim of science was to obtain knowledge so that we could dominate and control nature: "She must be bound."

However, over the years since the seventeenth century, we've learned that disease needs to be considered from the internal bioregulatory systems perspective as well as with an energetic and emotional angle. Fortunately, the role of the mind in medicine has slowly regained its place. The fields of psychoneuroimmunology and neuroimmunomodulation trace the pathways between emotions and disease, whose connections have long been viewed in clinical contexts by physicians ranging from Galen to Freud.[15] Neuroscientist Candace Pert, in her groundbreaking book, *Molecules of Emotion*, published in 1999, found that certain proteins called peptides (including endorphins) are among the body's key information substances that affect our mind, our emotions, our immune system, our digestion, and other bodily functions. Her research disproved Descartes, who insisted the mind and body be split—the body belonging to science and the mind to metaphysics.

But let's go back for just a moment. In the seventeenth century, when scientist Isaac Newton cast a mathematical, materialistic, and reductionist view upon the world, the body was seen as a machine, as

was everything else during that time of the Industrial Revolution—
a machine that was best understood if taken apart, with the very
smallest pieces analyzed. Descartes had already removed the mind
from medicine, and with Newton's reductionist theory, medicine
shifted to the perspective that organs and tissues should be viewed
in isolation, ignoring the whole. Medicine moved from the macro
to the micro, and therefore the quest to understand the body and
disease became more myopic. It was perfect timing for microbiology to enter the scene.

In the late 1800s, what was perhaps the best-known medical
feud raged between two French scientists: Louis Pasteur, who
discovered the science of microbiology and suggested the theory
that microorganisms were the basis of disease, and his rival, scientist Antoine Beauchamp, who disagreed with this simplistic germ
theory, suggesting that the "biological terrain" (the body's internal
environment) was more important than microbes. The germ/
gene cause of disease became the foundation of allopathy, while
imbalances in the terrain as the root of disease established the base
camp of BioMed and many other natural medicine modalities.
But Pasteur's theory won the popular vote, despite the fact that
Beauchamp's underreceived claim was reinforced with the seed and
soil hypothesis asserted in 1889 by Stephen Paget. Paget found that
some cancerous tumor cells—what he referred to as the "seed"—
grew preferentially in the microenvironment of select organs, which
he called the "soil." Paget theorized that metastases resulted only
when the appropriate seeds were implanted in suitable soils and
the microenvironment (the terrain) supported their growth. Simply,
two people could be exposed to the same germs and have the same
cancer cells in their body, but only one might get sick because of
the state of their terrain. Interestingly, when Pasteur was on his
deathbed, he is anecdotally reported to have said that Bernard was
right, "*Le germe n'est rien, c'est le terrain qui est tout*"—"The microbe
is nothing, the soil is everything."[16]

Regardless of this, the seed and soil theory was cast to the wind
as nineteenth-century medicine was infected with the germ theory.
With the dawn of bacteriology, the development of immunizations,

pasteurization, and antibiotics (which means "anti-life") accelerated at a dizzying pace from the late 1800s through the 1930s. And why not? It made sense to a world that was reeling from the flu pandemic of 1889 that killed a million people while malaria continued to scourge the globe. It was time for answers, and fast. It was also a time during which money and medicine fell deeply in love. And when that happened, all alternative schools of thought were closed, cast aside, discredited, and banished in favor of the conventional allopathic drug-based model.

There was actually one document that discredited all other medical sects aside from allopathy, called the *Flexner Report*, written by educator Abraham Flexner and published in 1910 under the sponsorship of the Carnegie and Rockefeller Foundations. The report called on American medical schools to enact higher admission and graduation standards, and to adhere strictly to the protocols of "mainstream" science in their teaching and research. The mainstream at the time was firmly planted in the world of microbiology; *holistic* was not part of their vocabulary. To Flexner, illegitimate "nonscientific" approaches in the medical marketplace, including the offerings of so-called folk psychologists, naturopaths, homoeopaths, chiropractors, and osteopaths, were actively competing with the modern conventional scientific paradigm of research and education. To him their models were "wrong," and therefore dangerous.[17] *Flexner's Report* subsequently led to shutting down the majority of complementary and alternative-oriented colleges and programs (medical schools, homoeopathic colleges, and some psychiatric institutions) before and after World War I. The remaining approved medical research and education programs were funded by philanthropic organizations such as the Rockefeller Foundation and the Carnegie Foundation; foundations that also had lots of money in the pockets of drug developers. These foundations and the *Flexner Report* fueled a medical coup against Hippocratic and holistic medicine, labeling them as quackery. Bulldozed by heavily funded bullies, natural medicine practitioners were shoved out of favor, making way for the new era of medicine: synthetic prescription pharmaceutical drugs.

Today's pharmaceutical companies were once apothecaries that transitioned into wholesale drug production in the middle of the nineteenth century. Merck, for example, began as a small apothecary shop in Darmstadt, Germany, in 1668, only beginning wholesale production of drugs in the 1840s. Then, dye and chemical companies established research labs and discovered medical applications for their products in the 1880s. Chemicals firms that morphed into pharmaceutical companies include Bayer and Pfizer. Those companies also established cooperative relationships with academic labs. The American Chemical Society's Division of Medicinal Chemistry was founded in 1909 and called the Division of Pharmaceutical Chemistry. Chemicals became synonymous with medicine, and the bonds were sealed among a treacherous trilogy: chemical, pharmaceutical, and educational. But amid the chemical drug development and research hysteria, there was another scientist playing around with some ideas. Ideas that would take the all-but-forgotten energy focus of ancient and Hippocratic medical models to a whole new frequency, keeping the heart of BioMed beating among the drums of industrialized medicine.

Einstein, Energy, and Quantum Theory

German-born theoretical physicist Albert Einstein changed the faces of both science and medicine forever in the early 1900s. In contrast with the body-is-mechanical Newtonian perspective, Einstein asserted that human beings are 100 percent energy. He said, "Everything is energy and that's all there is. Match the frequency of the reality you want and you cannot help but get that reality. It can be no other way. This is not philosophy. This is physics." Einstein was a pioneer in quantum theory, explaining the nature and behavior of matter and energy on an atomic and subatomic level. The cutting-edge field of energy medicine (which deeply influences bioregulatory medicine) is based on the fundamental premise that all physical objects (bodies) and psychological processes (thoughts, emotions, beliefs, and attitudes) are expressions of energy, and are not simply mechanistic. The quantum and energy theories of

Einstein bestowed a modern explanation to the ancients' views of energy—things like qi and *veda*. And as we will explore deeper throughout this book, energy *is* everything, and *is* the key to health and healing. Natural, biologically derived medicine contains energy, and energy is what is required to change the terrain.

Even in allopathic medicine there are many well-established uses of measurable energy fields in both the diagnosis and treatment of disease. Some of these include: magnetic resonance imaging (MRIs), laser eye correction surgery, cardiac pacemakers, radiation therapy, and UV light therapies for psoriasis and seasonal affective disorder. Yet the allopathic modality continues to focus solely on the biochemistry of cells, tissues, and organs, while energy medicine focuses on the body's energy fields that organize and control the growth and repair of cells, tissues, and organs. Repairing impaired energy patterns, bioregulatory systems, and mitochondria is the most efficient, least invasive way to improve the vitality of organs, cells, and psyche. This can only be done by changing energy through the use of energetic medicine found in naturally occurring elements. Thanks to Einstein, we know that our bodies, or our physical world, as well as our thoughts and beliefs are all part of a resonant field of vibrating, oscillating energy. And our energy is affected by our lifestyles, our environment, and our emotions. The ancient medical views that sustained human health for thousands of years were at last confirmed by Einstein's quantitative energy theories.

Energy medicine furthered its just accolades when Niels Ryberg Finsen (1860–1904), a Danish physician and scientist, was awarded the Nobel Prize in medicine and physiology in 1903 for his contribution to the treatment of diseases, especially lupus vulgaris, with concentrated light radiation. Radiation is the emission or transmission of energy in the form of waves or particles through space or a material medium. Visible light is a form of electromagnetic radiation, as are radio waves, infrared radiation, ultraviolet radiation, X-rays, and microwaves. Cancer radiation therapy, for example, uses a special kind of high-energy beam to damage cancer cells, which is actually a form of energy medicine using light, or *photons* (based on the Greek word for light). Each photon contains energy.

German biophysicist Fritz-Albert Popp (born in 1938) proved that light in our body is actually stored by, and emitted from, our DNA. We knew that plants used energy from sunlight to make food, but it became clear that plants are not the only living beings that have a complex relationship with and need for light; the biophotons emitted from human DNA, in fact, regulate the activity of metabolic enzymes. We know today that man is basically a beam of light. When a cell dies the process looks very similar under a microscope to the death of a star. As genius Nikola Tesla, electrical engineer, physicist, and futurist, said, "If you want to find the secrets of the universe think in terms of energy, frequency and vibration."

Bioregulatory medicine sees humans as a triangle of health that is biophysiological, energetic, and emotional. Referred to in other paradigms as meridian points, chakras, veda, or qi, energy has been officially "validated" by modern science. Energy medicine, until recently, has been largely disregarded by the mainstream, yet it is the most innovative, safe, and effective form of medicine. Today—through proven research—modern medicine has bestowed a name to these energetic influences: biofields. The term *biofield* was coined in the early 1990s by the National Institutes of Health as: "a massless field, not necessarily electromagnetic, that surrounds and permeates living bodies and affects the body."[18] A biofield (also called a biological field) is a human's complex organizing energy field that is involved in the generation, maintenance, and regulation of biophysiological homodynamics. All living systems are controlled by our biofields (energy), which have been scientifically proven to influence a variety of biophysiological pathways, including biochemical, cellular, and neurological processes. These biofields include energy and information that actually surround and interpenetrate the human body, holding and conveying intelligence that is vital for bioregulation. Biofield science is an emerging field of study aiming to provide a scientific foundation for understanding the complex homodynamic regulation of living systems. But this is something we humans have known for a long time; it was called "vital force" about three thousand years ago. Of course, from an allopathic perspective, under the assumption that "life is chemistry," energy medicine, or the application of extremely low-level signals to the body via bio-electromagnetic device-based therapies, is incomprehensible.[19] It's time to change that view. Energy medicine focuses on refueling and repairing mitochondria, giving needed fuel to cells to help facilitate bioregulation. These nontoxic treatments, including electron foot-baths, oxygen therapies, electromagnetic vibration, and bioresonance therapy, are all tools used by bioregulatory medical providers.

Have you seen how singers can shatter a wineglass by hitting and sustaining the correct note? Glass has a specific resonant frequency, which is the speed at which it will vibrate if disturbed by a stimulus such as a sound wave. What's more, every material on Earth has its own resonant frequency, just as Einstein asserted. Based on this idea, the infamous (and controversial) microbiologist Royal Raymond Rife (1888–1971) discovered a cancer therapy he called resonance therapy. His Rife machine was based on a naval radio frequency oscillator, and it destroyed pathogens, bacteria, viruses, and cancer cells using high-frequency energies created by electronic equipment. His machine could shatter biological living organisms like a crystal glass. Rife figured out that a specific resonant frequency would cause a microorganism to oscillate, or swing back and forth. By turning up the intensity, he could cause the structural integrity of the microorganism, such as a virus, to collapse and destroy itself. Rife called this phenomenon the mortal oscillatory rate, or MOR. Sadly, the American medical establishment silenced him, but his work lives on. Watch the TED Talk by Anthony Holland, associate professor and director of music technology at Skidmore College, titled, "Shattering Cancer with Resonant Frequencies." Ask your doctor about this if you have Lyme disease, MRSA, or cancer, as this type of therapy is part of the multimodal approach in bioregulatory medicine and is what makes it so effective.

DNA, Disconnect, and Fear

The nail in the coffin of disconnecting people from their health—especially on an emotional and spiritual plane—came with the discovery of DNA by Watson and Crick in the 1950s. They concluded that DNA "controls" the structure and behavior of living organisms and that all of our traits and characteristics are defined at the moment of conception. This hypothesis imparts a fatalistic view, disempowering individuals from their health, and has many people believing that their genes are in control. Yet genes don't actually cause the majority of diseases. In fact, one way disease can surface is by how genes respond to their environment, a modifiable response known as epigenetics. But this genes-and-germs-are-the-cause-of-illness mentality is why we are no closer to a cure against cancer and other chronic degenerative diseases than we were in the 1930s. Allopathic medicine and its philosophies have been trying to shove a square peg into the round hole of health for centuries, at the expense of the patient.

Since the end of the sixteenth century mainstream medicine has tried to take a very different road from the holistic, mind-body, and nature cure approach that has been with humankind for more than six thousand years and was lost in favor of an empiric, "prove it" mentality, along with a genetic and pathological lens. From a mainstream medicine perspective, unless a scientific, double-blind study proves something "works," there is no evidence to justify it to medical practitioners. Just ask your primary care provider if they think nutrition is an important part of a healing process, and more often than not the answer is (incorrectly) "there is not enough evidence to prove it." Meanwhile, drug companies are paying huge amounts of money to fund drug research to help "prove" their efficacy. The question of bias is too large for a book like this. But it's pretty simple: Whoever funds the study has a hand in the results. A January 2010 study in the *Journal of the American Medical Association* (*JAMA*) estimated that US medical research currently stands at over $100 billion annually and the pharmaceutical industry is the largest contributor toward research, funding over 60 percent. Is this transparent, patient-centered medicine?

Meanwhile, disease is not what it used to be. The rate of infectious diseases has been eclipsed by an epidemic of modern multifactorial chronic illnesses. Yet the drug-developing allopathic medicine model hasn't evolved to match the new epidemic. The word *doctor* is derived from the Latin word *docere*, meaning "to teach" or "to educate." As such, one of the primary responsibilities in bioregulatory medicine is to educate the patient and encourage self-responsibility for health. A cooperative doctor-patient relationship is essential for full healing. In bioregulatory medicine, patients are not passive, but are active participants in restoring their health and well-being—through nutritional modifications, lifestyle assessments, and managing their emotional landscapes (both past and present).

It is important for readers to know that there is no "quick fix" with bioregulatory medicine. With chronic and degenerative illnesses, true healing is often a long project. It's a marathon, not a sprint, and the patient has to do some of the running. This is hard for some people to swallow in an age of get-healthy-quick schemes that, though usually not an actual cure, give a false promise that *sounds* good. The bioregulatory medicine patient needs to have a long view about their health, for true healing can take years to achieve, followed by a lifetime of attention in order to remain at a place of optimal performance. It is important to understand that optimal performance doesn't mean someone will *never* get sick, but rather that the person will be in a place to recover from illness in as short a time as possible. As such, prevention, which means living in accordance with natural laws, is the key to maintaining optimal performance. Yet if a chronic or degenerative disease has grabbed hold of you, don't abandon hope. In bioregulatory medicine, there is no such thing as an incurable disease. Our bodies, as we have discussed, have an innate ability to heal. Healing is what our bioregulatory systems are designed to do. So let's dive deeper into these systems that are hard at work keeping you healthy and examine the ways we can assess them. Get ready, because there is a whole lot more to health than you might realize.

Bioregulatory Medicine
The Future of Health and Healing

The noblest foundation for medicine is love. It is love which teaches us the art of healing. Without love, true healing cannot be born.

—PARACELSUS

The good physician treats the disease; the great physician treats the patient who has the disease.

—SIR WILLIAM OSLER

A s we now know, the role of bioregulatory medicine practitioners is to identify and remove whatever agents are blocking the healing process while helping to restore the body's innate ability to rehabilitate and regenerate. We also know that healing cannot be achieved if we don't correctly identify what the root cause of the imbalance is. We know that treating and assessing the whole person is directed at both underlying and immediate causative factors while also recognizing the interconnectivity between physical and nonphysical components of the human body. We know that someone could seem physically healthy, but an unstable emotional environment can have a negative impact on their terrain and be a precursor to future illness. With BioMed, we have a new view of health and disease and the factors that influence it.

Like a log that has fallen across a flowing river, at the root of most illnesses are psycho-emotional and environmental toxic blockades that overwhelm the body's regulatory systems. Consider a barrel that is filling with water. Every stressful event, every bite of toxic food, every exposure to mercury fillings is akin to pouring more water in that barrel. With every drop, more symptoms appear. Once the barrel is full it overflows into a disease state. But while everyone has a barrel, the influencing factors that fill each barrel are unique to each person. We all have different life stressors, dietary habits, thought processes, past traumas, and environments. Each person, depending on their emotional type or miasm (inherited predispositions toward physical and/or mental illnesses or weaknesses), also adapts in his or her own way to these barrel-filling factors. To one person, getting stuck in traffic is maddening, and it fills their disease barrel a little bit. To another, traffic allows more relaxation time to listen to a favorite book on tape, and therefore it doesn't add water to their barrel. How a person reacts—regulates—in response to causal factors is in part due to genetic predisposition, emotional/mental characteristics, bioenergetic factors, social circumstances, and more. How full the barrel gets over the years plays an important role in the development of chronic illness. This is a process that might appear suddenly or insidiously, slowly mounting over months or even years. At the end of the day, both health and disease result from a complex interaction and reaction to physical, mental, emotional, environmental, genetic, spiritual, and social factors. A harmonious functioning and the ability to properly respond to all these dysregulating aspects is the blueprint to health.

The term *regulation capacity* is a measurement of a person's ability to react. It essentially refers to how many pushes one can take and still remain regulated or balanced. When the body is in balance, it is not as prone to chronic illness, and it remains in a state of health, or homeostasis. Regulation is about reaction. If you throw a ball at someone's face, they should react by either trying to catch the ball or dodging it so they don't get hit. If a light turns on, the iris constricts in the eye. If someone gets bitten by a Lyme-carrying tick, their body's autoregulating systems—immune, digestive, and inflammatory—need to react against the bacteria. Reaction is regulation, regulation is adaptation, and the ability to regulate is *the* key to health. But if a person's barrel is too full or there are too many logs blocking their flowing river, then regulation and reaction cannot happen. The body slows, cells degenerate, and we run out of energy. Too much energy has been expended trying to get back to homeostasis.

Chronic disease occurs when a person has a lowered regulation capacity to such an extent that inherent healing forces are no longer able to react against disease-causing conditions with their normal and usual corrective efforts. Disease—quite simply—is a reduced regulation capacity. Regulation capacity is how well a person can adapt and react, and regulation logjams are what trigger or worsen chronic diseases. Bioregulatory medicine looks to remove the logjams and drain the barrel, all of which allow the resources for self-healing mechanisms to grow stronger, permitting self-healing to happen.

The terms *self-heal* and *regenerate* both refer to the self-repair forces inherent to humans. We know the body has the ability to regenerate, as our tissues regenerate all the time (think of a cut on your finger turning into a scab, then healing over completely). Over a life span, our body grows, develops, matures, and declines. Within this cycle of life, every one of the body's cells and organs has its own regeneration cycle. Some cells are programmed to die after forty or so divisions. Every organ in the body has a regeneration cycle where old cells die and new cells are generated. Intestinal bacteria regenerate within several days, the intestinal wall within two weeks, and immune cells within four weeks. The liver possesses an extraordinary capacity to regenerate. As little as 25 percent of an original liver mass can regenerate back to its full size within six months. In general, the organs that do the most work encountering the outside world have the fastest regeneration rate. For example, the digestive lining and immune system cells have a far shorter life span than our bone, heart, and brain cells. Healing, therefore, depends on a tissue's regeneration time.

The default state of the body is one of ceaseless regeneration. In fact, every atom and molecule of the entire human body is replaced every seven to ten years without us even thinking about it. This is a natural process that requires no medical intervention. However, in chronic and degenerative disease this renewal process goes haywire. In the case of cancer, cells become immortal and are constantly dividing and growing. In degenerative nerve diseases such as Alzheimer's, cells of the nervous system degenerate instead of regenerate; they rot and die without replacement. Those following an allopathic medical track for neurodegenerative diseases end up on drugs such as dopamine antagonists and antiseizure medications that reduce the symptoms but don't stop the root of the problem: nerve degeneration. A bioregulatory medicine treatment approach is in stark contrast. We know that there are several natural and non-toxic compounds with proven nerve-regenerative effects, including Huperzine, Apigenin, and lion's mane mushroom, for example.[1] These phytochemicals stimulate the regenerative process, promote quality and quantity of life, and shoot to cure.

The BioMed Patient Assessment

Bioregulatory medical providers take a patients' medical history on their first appointment, like any conventional general practitioner (GP) would do. But the similarities generally stop there. Bioregulatory medicine therapists focus also on a comprehensive multisystem psychological and bioenergetic assessment; structural evaluation, analysis of nutritional deficiencies, toxicities, childhood traumas, and beyond in order to identify the dysregulatory factors involved in the process of symptoms or pathology. Allopathic GPs ask about symptoms, specific complaints, and review basic serum lab tests in order to match them with a diagnosis code and a prescription. Bioregulatory doctors, by contrast, think in patterns and connections and consider the patient's story. For bioregulatory doctors, it is not about the diagnosis but rather about the systems at play. In the art of the bioregulatory intake, there is an element of intuition, where practitioners have learned to recognize, for example, that adverse events in childhood can manifest into pathology later in life. For example, if during adolescence certain coping strategies for psycho-emotional issues are not learned, addictive behavior can manifest in adulthood. Multiple food intolerances in early childhood can present later in life in immune system deficiencies or digestive or pulmonary issues. Those with toxin exposure in their past might present with cancer in the future. It's all about recognizing cause and effect, the factors filling the barrel. Disease doesn't just show up on your doorstep one day, just as (most) marriages don't end in divorce in one day. Disease is *never* bad luck.

While the primary diagnostic tools of a bioregulatory medicine practitioner include those of any other physician—lab tests, blood work, X-rays, scans, scopes, histories, and physicals—the bioregulatory medicine practitioner also employs additional tools so they can examine each patient on multiple levels. These tools include, but are not limited to:

- Physical body examination and constitution analysis
- Dental examination and panoramic X-ray
- Organ biocommunication scans
- General blood work, including orthomolecular
- Genetic and SNP analysis testing
- Body composition analysis
- Dark field microscopy
- Hormone testing
- Heavy-metal testing (urine/blood/hair analysis)
- Intestinal flora and comprehensive stool analysis
- Food intolerances (IgA, IgG, IgG4)
- Heart rate variability (HRV)
- Contact regulation thermography (CRT)

Using the most technologically advanced diagnostic testing allows the bioregulatory medical provider to perform a core tenet: *tolle causam*, or identify and treat the cause. Bioregulatory medicine employs noninvasive diagnostic aids that view not only structural imbalances, but also functional, metabolic, genetic, regulatory, energetic, and psycho-emotional conditions. Hence, environmental toxins, lifestyle, social and professional influences, and ecological terrain and genetic information are all vital factors to evaluate. If a patient walks in with dermatitis, instead of simply prescribing a steroid cream, the bioregulatory medical practitioner will seek out the root cause of that inflammation—a food sensitivity, poor kidney or liver function, impaired oxygenation, weak lung activity, stress at work, or a combination thereof. The symptom is usually the end result of an imbalance in several systems. Lots of pushes off the beam, the barrel overflowing, the river clogged with logs.

Illness does not occur without a cause, and symptoms (nausea, vomiting, headache, rash, fever, etc.) are not the cause of illness. As we have discussed, symptoms are an expression of the body's attempt to defend itself, to adapt and recover, and to heal. When symptoms are treated via palliation and suppression (allopathically), and the underlying causes are ignored, the patient might develop a more serious, chronic condition. Etiologies, or causes of disease, usually exist simultaneously. Disease develops in a causal chain, one begetting the other. Bioregulatory medical providers not only discover the primary cause of the illness, but also identify the weakest afflicted organ or system. This is called the causal chain—which is essentially a flow chart that represents the evolution of the pathological history of the patient, taking into account all the possible manifestations and the evolution of a disease.

Treatment on the Terrain (or Internal Milieu)

Bioregulatory medicine sees imbalances in the biological terrain as the root of disease. For example, *Streptococcus* is not viewed as the cause of strep throat, but rather as a breakdown in the body's immune system that then creates a hospitable environment for this gram-positive bacteria to transform into an infectious and virulent form. An allopathic medicine treatment plan would kill the *Streptococcus* with antibiotics and suppress the associated fever with aspirin. From a bioregulatory medicine perspective, fever is the body's natural response to stimulate the immune system and should not be suppressed; rather the biological terrain should be supported through rest, hydrotherapy, herbs, vitamins, probiotics, and so on.

To back up for a moment, the *internal terrain* or *milieu* is a conceptual term coined by nineteenth-century French physician Claude Bernard and refers to the internal environment of an organism.

Any type of disturbance of the balance between the cells and the surrounding cell milieu can lead to a functional disorder and later to cellular degeneration or cancer. Our organs, glands, and tissue cells are embedded in a complex bioregulatory extracellular matrix (ECM) consisting of water, proteins, carbohydrates, and fats. It is in the ECM that the causes and cures of many of the so-called systemic and chronic illnesses, especially inflammatory conditions, are most appropriately addressed. And it is also in the ECM that many of the biologically oriented therapeutics exert their effect. All nutritional substances—oxygen, vitamins, minerals—reach the cell by passing through this matrix. Therefore cellular detoxification, communication, and regeneration are dependent upon the health and integrity of the bioregulatory matrix.

Various influencing factors can destroy and dysregulate the matrix and, thus, the biosphere of the cells. Repair of tissue after physical or chemical injury depends on the synthesis of the ECM to replace lost or damaged tissue. The ECM directs repair by regulating the behavior of the wide variety of cell types that are mobilized to the damaged area to rebuild the tissue. Acute inflammation, reepithelialization, and contraction all depend on ECM interactions and contribute to minimizing toxicity and infection and promoting healing. So we see, and will continue to see, that BioMed embraces terrain-focused medical interventions in all cases of chronic and degenerative disease. Our health is more than just a medical construct, it is a reflection of how we choose to live. Humans cannot achieve optimal levels of health living in unhealthy environments, while eating toxic foods or not getting enough rest or exercise. It is the responsibility of the physician to make the patient aware of these factors. It is then the patient's responsibility to create an environment that will be conducive to health and supportive of the body's internal milieu. There are many factors that can adversely impact the biological terrain, including:

- Dehydration
- Food allergies
- Improper diet and overeating

- Stress
- Heavy metals and environmental toxins
- Dental problems
- Vaccinations
- Medications
- Hidden infections
- Lack of exercise
- Electromagnetic field (EMF) exposure
- Lack of sunlight
- Structural imbalances and injury

All these factors can be prevented. Recall one of the core principles of bioregulatory medicine of utilizing the healing power of nature, or *vis medicatrix naturae*. Reverend Sebastian Kneipp (1821–97), a Bavarian priest and one of the forefathers of bioregulatory medicine, cured himself from tuberculosis using natural methods. At that time the disease was usually fatal, but Kneipp learned about the ancient wisdom of using water as a means of therapy. He decided to immerse himself several times a week in the frigid Danube River. These brief exposures to cold water bolstered his immune system enough to send his disease into remission. Heat and cold, dryness and moisture, light and air, as well as proper nutrition, are all part of the traditions of Hippocrates and are the important cornerstones of bioregulatory medicine today.

Ask a room full of people what they think causes illness. Germs is generally the most common answer, followed by genes, toxins, diet, and stress. But the real cause of illness is violations against natural laws. German medical doctor Henry Lindlahr was the author of one of the cornerstone texts of bioregulatory medicine, *Nature Cure*. The book includes topics such as disease suppression versus elimination, hydrotherapy, and the importance of fresh air and sunbathing. It was inspired by his own healing journey alongside his mentor, cold-plunger Kneipp. The reasons why *Nature Cure* is not popular within the allopathic medical profession and the public are twofold: First, it is just too simple. But also, it is drugless healing, which means pharmaceutical companies can't profit from it. Bioregulatory practitioners recognize that if their patients are not living in accordance with natural laws to start, then health or healing will not be attained.

Today, in small corners, using various natural cures has become hip and trendy, but it's been given a new name: bio-hacking. This do-it-yourself, improve-your-biology trend has become a social movement, where people have found that adapting natural law "tricks" such as fasting or spending at least thirty minutes a day outside, no matter what the weather, can improve their health and cognitive performance. These natural law tricks include outdoor time in extreme temperatures, exercising, sleeping, staying hydrated (most people with chronic illness are dehydrated), eating whole foods, playing, laughing, meditating, and breathing. All of these activities, either individually or done in tandem, have been shown to have a positive impact on healing chronic diseases, from depression to colon cancer. Living in accordance with natural laws is the prescription for prevention that bioregulatory medicine teaches all patients—no matter where they are on the health continuum. It's time to start changing the health and disease stories of our loved ones and ourselves. And this prescription is not just about curing chronic illnesses; medicine should be about health promotion and community—*that* is the future of medicine. BioMed is not a new or fringy idea and to learn about just a few of the BioMed pioneers, we primarily look overseas to Europe.

The Origins of BioMed

Bioregulatory medicine got its modern start in Germany during the early 1900s. In 1905, Dr. F. Bachmann united many like-minded physicians together in the Biological Medicine Society (Medizinisch-biologische Gesellschaft), which promoted biological regulatory medicine at conferences in Hamburg in 1912, and Dresden in 1924. At the turn of the nineteenth century, many doctors were still practicing homeopaths and many of those homeopaths were also Jewish. In Germany and throughout Europe, World War I and World War II brought chaos and destroyed much of the bioregulatory medicine movement (which, as we discussed in the introduction, was referred to as European Biological Medicine). During World War II many Jewish scientists and homeopaths fled Germany for North and South America. It was not until the end of the National Socialist regime in the mid-1940s that a new renaissance in biological regulatory medicine started in Germany, Austria, and Switzerland, transitioning into what is today simply called bioregulatory medicine.

There are more than fifty pioneering contributors to the herbal, nutritional, homeopathic, energetic, and dental arms of bioregulatory medicine who were born before 1910. It would take a whole book to tell all of their tales of medical innovations and discoveries. Saint Hildegard of Bingen (1098–1179), for example, was an abbess, mystic, healer, visionary, and herbalist who believed God had given mankind herbs, spices, and foods to serve our bodies and keep us healthy. She authored two major medical treatises outlining nine categories of healing systems: plants, elements, trees, stones, fish, birds, animals, reptiles, and metals. These papers were the foundations of natural medicine. Due to her outstanding work, which unfortunately no one was able to understand at that time, she was later made a saint in the Roman Catholic Church.

Christoph Wilhelm Friedrich Hufeland was a German physician born in 1762, and *Makrobiotik* was his masterpiece on preventive medicine. First published in 1797, the book had eight official editions appearing during his lifetime and several translations. The organizing principle for understanding human life and health in *Makrobiotik* was the life force (called *lebenskraft*). This life force, according to Hufeland, is manifested in organic beings as the ability to respond to external stimuli. He believed that this force could be weakened or destroyed, as well as strengthened, through external influences. *Lebenskraft* is depleted through bodily exertion and increased with rest. Hufeland believed that moral and physical health were intertwined and flowing from the same life force. The concept of life force has clearly been present for a very, very long time.

Constantine Hering, one of the giants of homeopathy, was born on January 1, 1800, in Oschatz, Germany. He authored a number of books, including *The Guiding Symptoms of Our Materia Medica*, which was based on fifty years of his research. Hering was involved with proving over ninety remedies and also founded the first homeopathic schools in the United States. Among his many contributions to the medical field were his observations of the healing process, coined Hering's Law of Cure, the way the body acts to heal itself. Hering formulated the law based on observed that the body seeks to externalize disease, noting that symptoms will surface as part of the curative process (e.g., rashes), and a person's symptoms will appear and disappear in the reverse order of their appearance upon the body. Thus, a patient might reexperience symptoms during the healing process as the body heals from top to bottom, and from more vital organs to less vital organs. Today we call this a healing crisis—when people tend to feel a bit worse before they feel better. Just ask anyone who has ever done a two-week cleanse how they felt on the third day.

At the end of the eighteenth century and the early nineteenth century, we saw the advent of several distinct natural healing fields that are also considered limbs on the tree of bioregulatory medicine. These include osteopathic, chiropractic, holistic dentistry, and elements of psychological medicine. Carl Gustav Jung (1876–1961) was a Swiss psychiatrist who emphasized the important role of the unconscious mind. Wilhelm Reich (1897–1957) was an Austrian psychoanalyst who discovered a form of energy he called "orgone" and asserted that this energy could be found within all living things and throughout the cosmos. One of Reich's books, *Character Analysis*, published in 1933, was groundbreaking. It suggested that a person's overall character, rather than only their symptoms, should be considered when diagnosing and analyzing neurosis.

Canadian-born dentist Weston A. Price (1870–1948) researched the relationship between nutrition, dental health, and physical health. Price developed the theory that systemic conditions including intestinal disorders and anemia were caused by infections in the mouth. In 1925 he published the book *Dental Infections and Related Degenerative Diseases*. Price also founded the National Dental Association and pioneered the holistic dentistry movement. It is worth noting that medicine and dentistry were one and the same until the mid-1800s. As medicine began to demand specialists, oral care was divorced from medicine's education systems and payment systems. Today a dentist is not just a different kind of doctor but is considered another profession entirely. Of course our *teeth* don't know that they're supposed to keep their problems confined to the mouth. Still the connections proven between location of dental infection and location of organ dysfunctions, including breast cancer, cannot be ignored.

Also in the late 1800s, when allopathic medicine was looking at cancer treatment with a chemical-warfare lens, those in the bioregulatory medicine field were discovering and using other highly effective yet nontoxic approaches. These BioMed treatments had promising and prevailing results. Nobel Prize–winning German Otto Heinrich Warburg (1883–1970) discovered that cancer cells had an altered metabolism, and were low in oxygen due to a change in their cellular respiration. Warburg's discovery is the foundation of the metabolic hallmark of cancer that is gaining major modern traction in both drug development and dietary interventions today. Around the same time, Austrian Rudolf Joseph Lorenz Steiner (1861–1925) and Indonesian/Dutch Ita Wegman (1876–1943) cofounded a spiritual science called anthroposophical medicine, a belief that everything physical is infused with and manifests spirit—the earliest hint at epigenetics. Steiner and Wegman also developed a natural immunotherapy treatment using an extract of mistletoe. The remedy, called *Iscador*, has been an approved and effective cancer treatment in Germany and a number of other countries for decades and is currently undergoing clinical trials in the United States. Sadly, Americans who can afford it have, to date, had to travel overseas to cancer clinics in countries such as Switzerland in order to have access to mistletoe therapy.

Finally, an American entered the scene. William Bradley Coley (1862–1936), a bone surgeon and pioneer of cancer immunotherapy, injected the *Streptococcus* bacteria into a terminal cancer patient, eliciting a high fever that subsequently dissolved an inoperable tumor. This was a medical miracle. (The healing miracle of a fever, which bioregulatory doctors had been using for centuries.) Isn't it amazing that, even after Coley's medical miracle, Western medicine continued to suppress the power of fever with use of bioengineered immunotherapy substances? Also in the cancer realm was Josef M. Issels (1907–98), a German physician who was dedicated to treating advanced and standard therapy-resistant cancers. Known for promoting an alternative cancer therapy regimen that he named the Issels treatment, his therapies included detoxification; nutritional support; supplementation with vitamins, minerals, and enzymes; chelation therapy; acupuncture; massage therapy; counseling; oxygen/ozone therapy; vaccines; and light therapy. Issels's methods were truly integrated, natural, polytherapy, bioregulatory approaches to treating cancer and chronic illness.

What we see is that these nature cure treatments and concepts are focused on the terrain. Once we go deeper into the terrain, the wonders of the body's bioregulating systems that create and sustain life become illuminated. Successful medicine, bioregulatory medicine, is focused on using treatments that encourage the harmonious functioning and homeostasis of all these systems. In the next chapter we will discuss each of these systems and introduce a few of the diagnostics and treatments used to assess and address each one.

Implementing a Systems-Based Approach to Bioregulation, Regeneration, and Healing

Natural forces within us are the true healers of disease.

—HIPPOCRATES

When we recognise the virtues, the talent, the beauty of Mother Earth, something is born in us, some kind of connection; love is born.

—THICH NHAT HANH

S imilar to (and fortunately for) humans, the Earth's self-regulating biosphere creates an environment suitable for our survival. Ceaseless geological and biological cycles create elements required for life—compounds such as water, carbon, nitrogen, and oxygen. These natural biocycles balance and regulate the Earth's habitable spaces. Take photosynthesis, for example: the sunlight-fueled oxygen- and energy-creation process required for human existence. Humans can't live without oxygen. Think about the water cycle: Clouds form over the ocean because oceanic algae emit sulfur molecules that become the condensation nuclei required for raindrop formation. Humans can't live without water. All combined, the many ecosystems on our planet—the land, the sea, and the atmosphere—are considered one self-sustaining unit. One biosphere. We humans have evolved to inhabit a planet where each ecosystem has its own set of regulatory processes—therefore, so do we.

Considering our multitude of bioregulating systems, the human body is largely a reflection of the Earth. Both are approximately 70 percent water, both require energy to sustain life, and both have their own set of bioregulatory cycles designed to keep them alive. Humans have a multitude of survival-dependent, symbiotic relationships with the planet. We depend on bees for food, microbes for immunity, trees and plankton for oxygen, lakes and rivers for water. Our respiratory system breathes the correct amount of oxygen into the body; the cardiovascular system then distributes the oxygen through the blood. Our digestive system converts food into energy. From a bioregulatory medicine lens, there is no denying the interconnection between humans and our planet. How could we be separate from or attempt to control our environment through man-made means? None of us are synthetic.

The Gaia theory (Gaia was the ancient Greek goddess of the Earth) was originally developed in the late 1960s by Dr. James Lovelock, a British scientist, inventor, and NASA staffer. The theory posits that the organic and inorganic components of planet Earth evolved together as a single living, self-regulating system. It suggests that Earth is a living system that automatically controls global temperature, atmospheric content, and ocean salinity in order to maintain its own habitability. It's not a stretch to compare the living systems of Earth to the interconnected workings of human bioregulatory systems, and how we self-modulate our body temperature, blood salinity, blood pressure, heart rate, and so on. We simply cannot separate ourselves from the environment, despite Western medicine's dismissal of interconnectedness. Just ask anyone who has lived through a powerful hurricane, wildfire, or other natural disaster who the boss is, because it's certainly not humans. We are a part of the whole, and many systems come together to keep the whole healthy. All life on Earth requires a complex and interdependent system of feedback loops that react to information from the environment. Each input into the system causes a change in homeostasis that requires a reaction to rebalance it. To maintain homeostasis, a complex and coordinated set of biochemical, thermal, and neural factors interact between every system in the body and also the environment. A primary element of the human body's homeostasis is largely controlled by the planet and our rhythmic responses to it.

The Earth-Health Connection: The Essence of Biorhythms

Every single day, 365 days a year, self-sustained and genetically programmed oscillations in behavior, physiology, and metabolism occur in all living beings on Earth, including humans, plants, animals, fungi, and cyanobacteria. Referred to as biorhythms (from Greek βίος—*bios*, meaning "life," and *rhuthmos*, meaning "any regular recurring motion, rhythm"), they occur in response to tidal, circadian, weekly, monthly, seasonal, and annual cycles. Biological rhythm or biorhythm is an inherent harmony between humans and nature, and our bodies' responses to these rhythms allow us to adapt to Earth's environment. Brain-wave activity, hormone production, cell regeneration, and other biological activities change throughout approximate 24-hour, 30-day, 90-day, and 365-day periods. For example, in the endocrine system, the pineal gland (which is the primary circadian clock in mammals) produces increased melatonin (the sleep hormone) as the sun sets and the retina of the eye perceives fewer light pulses. When the sun rises, cortisol (the hormone that wakes us up) is produced by the adrenal glands. Interfering with circadian rhythms—which is technically interfering with natural law—leads to dysregulation and, eventually, disease. Research has proven that destruction of biological rhythms might accelerate the onset of multiple diseases, inducing Alzheimer's disease, cardiovascular disease, obesity, diabetes, and metabolic syndromes, and is a risk factor for cancer development.[1] While modern "prove-it" research on this topic is infantile, recognition of the health-biorhythm connection is primordial. In fact, observations of various biorhythmic processes in humans are mentioned in Chinese medical texts dating back to the thirteenth century.

Body temperature varies during the course of the day, and also changes during ovulation in the menstrual cycle. Just ask a healthy menstruating woman how often she gets her period—a regular cycle is roughly once every month. Approximately one month is the time interval that the Moon takes to orbit 360 degrees around the Earth. Changes to metabolism are seen also with seasonal variation—every ninety days or so. Seasonal changes in food availability used to be the given—and our genetic controls of these biorhythms adapted as such. For example, the master fuel sensor in our cells during summer months is called mTOR (which stands for "mammalian target of rapamycin"). mTOR facilitates protein synthesis and growth while inhibiting the internal recycling of used or damaged cells. Things grow in summertime because there is more food and more light. Winter, until about three hundred years ago, used to be a time of caloric restriction, when resources stored from the summer and fall were consumed with great efficiency to ensure survival. The master fuel sensor in the winter is AMP-activated protein kinase (AMPK). AMPK optimizes energy efficiency and stimulates the recycling of cellular materials. This cycle also occurs to a lesser extent each night and during fasting. The pathways activated by AMPK support cellular regeneration and are also anti-inflammatory because they work to break down damaged proteins, lipids, glycans, RNA, and DNA.[2] We were designed to build muscle and fat in the summer and break it down in the winter. We had to. Consider the environmentally driven evolutionary forces that acted on our ancestors, who, up until a mere ten thousand years ago, did not have artificial light, a steady food supply, or temperature control. This might help to explain why people gain weight and get more colds and flus in the wintertime, they do not restrict their calories rather they increase them. (As tasty as it is, eggnog overload and sugar cookies are completely foreign to our genetics—especially in the wintertime.) You see, the body is in constant adaptation with our environment, both in the short term and in the long term. If we hadn't learned to adapt, we wouldn't have survived.

Whenever there is a season change, according to traditional Chinese medicine (TCM), the energy frequency of the body, or a person's qi, will change to match the season's frequency. TCM has always believed that each season has corresponding elements, organs, and emotions. Fall, for example, is associated with the lung and large intestine. When one's energy is not in tune during this time, illness, like the common cold with a cough, will appear. The lung is also associated with grief, and often that emotion will surface as we turn inward after a summer of outdoor expansion, when leaves die and fall to the ground. TCM has identified not only seasonal organ connections, but also the relationships between our organs and the twenty-four-hour cycle. For example, detoxification occurs between 1 a.m. and 3 a.m., when our livers are most active, and tissues and cells release toxins and acids. Nighttime is also when the repair-focused growth hormone is highest and cortisol levels are lowest. If someone is prone to waking during these hours, it is often a sign that the liver is congested. According to TCM, the bowels are most active between 5 a.m. and 7 a.m. when toxins that are released from the cells during sleep hours move into the colon. This is why we have morning breath, when urine smells the strongest, and bowel movements normally occur. Physiology is not coincidental.

It's not surprising that what TCM has known for thousands of years is now being verified by modern research. Studies have affirmed that more than 10 percent of expressed genes in all organs exhibit circadian oscillation.[3] In 2017, Jeffrey C. Hall, Michael Rosbash, and Michael W. Young won the Nobel Prize for their work identifying genetic mechanisms behind circadian rhythms—which adapt the workings of the body to different phases of the day, influencing sleep, behavior, hormone levels, body temperature, and metabolism. These clocks signal cells when to use energy, when to rest, and when to repair or replicate DNA. We now know that almost every cell in the body contains its own circadian clock. This biological timekeeping is actually a genetic process, one we share it with many bacteria, plants, animals, and even fungi. Also called peripheral oscillators, our cellular timekeepers have been found in the adrenal glands, lung, liver, pancreas, spleen, thymus, esophagus, and skin. These clock genes ensure the proper timing of metabolic events. Studies of clock-mutant mice—those who ate regardless of time of day—found increased obesity rates and altered glucose metabolism whereas those who ate within a smaller, eight-hour daylight window lost weight.[4] Our ancestors were not hunting and gathering in the dark—and therefore we shouldn't be eating at that time either. Chronic misalignment between our chosen modern lifestyle and the rhythms dictated by our inner timekeeper is associated with increased risk for various diseases, including cancer, degenerative neurological conditions, sleep disorders, depression, and bipolar disorder. The important takeaway is that our bodies are bioregulating systems that are influenced by our environment and its associated evolutionary genetic programming.

Understanding Our Life Cycle

Our bodies and organ systems develop and change over time following yet another cyclical pattern: our life cycle. The thymus gland, which helps to train important immune cells, including T cells, is largest and most active in newborns and infants and in the years prior to adolescence. But by the early teens the thymus begins to shrink and is replaced by fatty tissue. Over the course of a woman's life, for example, her ovaries will evolve from basic inactivity (birth to puberty), to increased production of estrogen (puberty), to regulating the monthly reproductive cycle (puberty until menopause), to eventually reducing production of estrogen as she enters menopause. We cannot underestimate the importance of physiological and energetic development and maturation of an organ system. In fact, the work of Rudolf Steiner, Ita Wegman, and others—currently being developed further by Dr. Dickson Thom— discovered that adult manifestations of specific diseases have roots in each life cycle. For example, the first phase of life is considered the adrenal phase, and includes the time between conception and eighteen months old. This is our survival phase, when fight or flight develops. Any type of trauma encountered during this phase, whether emotional, chemical, or physical, can manifest later as adrenal pathologies. By understanding the energetic maturation phases of organs, these stages can be returned to, and learned perceptions can be reprogramed. This process is how true healing occurs, by looking back at the energetic and physical phases of organ and system development and by reprogramming the body and mind with tools such as neurofeedback techniques, homeopathics, anthroposophical medicine, and more—all part of bioregulatory medicine.

How Did I Get Sick?

One of the most common questions patients ask their doctors when they are diagnosed is *why*. What caused the illness? The common allopathic medicine response is: *We don't really know*. That's just not good enough anymore, because we *do* know what causes disease: blocked and dysregulated bioregulatory systems that occur in response to our environment. Living outside of natural law, having a poor diet or unhealthy lifestyle, infections, toxic overload, and mental or emotional imbalances all disrupt systemic balance. Put twenty-five people who all have insomnia in a room and each will have their own causal factors, different than the others. Disease progression is an evolution that occurs over time and has roots in many physiological, biochemical, and emotional arenas. It is an absolute must in medicine to recognize the undeniable symbiosis between our health and our environment. Insomnia, for example, is a classic endocrine biorhythm dysregulation. Where allopathic medicine will throw highly addictive benzodiazepines at sleep issues, bioregulatory medicine will identify the bioregulatory blocking agents that are causing dysregulation of the melatonin and cortisol cycle and will stimulate and restore self-healing to the nervous and endocrine systems with biologically tuned treatments. Most people don't get to the point of lying awake all night for no reason—this dysregulation has identifiable roots and a causal chain. Bioregulatory medicine has identified just how disease evolves so that treatments can be tailored accordingly.

The Six Phases of Disease Evolution

Disease is the expression of the body's battle against dysregulations caused from numerous imbalances included but not limited to digestive distress, poor lymphatic function, inefficient detoxification, nutrient deficiencies, emotional distress, and oral imbalances. Therefore, it is important to assess the chronic disease process in a series of phases. For starters, we know that physiological health occurs when all bioregulatory systems are in balance. In health, when the body is exposed to external factors (physical, mental, or chemical), it will elicit an appropriate reaction to remove the external factor that might create symptoms, including various discharges and inflammation. At that point, internal compensation occurs, healthy function is reestablished, and symptoms vanish. The process is similar to how shock absorbers on your car withstand hardy potholes and keep you driving smoothly down the road. By the time we get to chronic and degenerative disease, the shocks are blown. Bioregulatory medicine has categorized disease evolution as a six-stage process.

The Excretion Phase

In the 1950s, German physician Hans-Heinrich Reckeweg combined ancient Chinese and naturopathic concepts to discern that illnesses are processes that have logical progression. According to Reckeweg, illnesses are agent-determined reactive processes in which homotoxins (substances that have a damaging effect on human cells) cause the body to react with inflammation. The first phase of disease development is called the excretion phase. Here the expulsion of toxins occurs through any tissue or organ capable of allowing excretions to exit the body, which are called emunctories. These include the kidneys and urinary tract, colon, lung, skin, and emotional brain. For this first phase, a good example is food poisoning and the immediate reaction of diarrhea or vomiting. Expulsion of toxins occurs immediately and normally through the physiological orifices. The body actively tries to rid the toxins from the body—that's a healthy response.

The Reaction Phase

The second phase is called the reaction phase, this phase is also when the body acts against dysregulating elements with an inflammatory response. Inflammation occurs to help mobilize white blood cells to destroy and remove the homotoxin. Inflammation—acute inflammation—is a protective bioregulating event. Thus, in the reaction phase the body might try to expel homotoxins with a fever. In fact, infections usually launch fever, especially in children. Other fever triggers include transfusion reactions, juvenile rheumatoid arthritis, tumors, inflammatory reactions caused by trauma, medications (including antihistamines, antibiotics, or an overdose of aspirin), immunizations, dehydration, and sometimes teething. In this phase defense mechanisms are active, providing valuable signs that the body is attempting to regulate toward recovery. Suppressing fevers and acute inflammations with allopathic drugs, such as NSAIDs or antifebrile medications, can further push dysregulation into a more advanced phase. In the reaction phase, the body *can* do what it needs to do to heal, but allopathic medicine is bent on stopping it.

Let's linger on the topic of fever for a moment. Fever occurs when infectious microorganisms stimulate white blood cells that then signal the brain's hypothalamus to raise the body's thermostat setting. In turn, fever heats the body by increasing its metabolic rate and immune activity. Given that most animals (vertebrates, anyway) mount a fever in response to illness, it's likely that humans have preserved this evolutionary response because it improves survival. Research supports this theory; animal studies show that when fever is blocked, survival rates from infection decline.[5] A fever has several purposes, including acting as a natural antibiotic: High temperatures can impair the replication of many bacteria and viruses and even destroy them. (This property is why we boil water to purify it.) Fever also causes thyroid stimulation, increasing basal metabolic rate, which aids the elimination of toxins. Suppressing a fever basically halts the action of the immune system and tells it to go on vacation. At temperatures higher than 105.5°F many of our body's proteins start to denature, and this is usually the time when we need to interfere not by taking a pill, rather by using alternatives such as cold wrappings to minimize the risk of possible cell damage. Bioregulatory medicine practitioners will support and monitor fevers where allopathic medicine practitioners suppress them—and there is a price for suppression.

The Deposition Phase

When fevers and acute inflammation fail to expel homotoxins, then the third phase of disease progression occurs, what's called the deposition phase. In the deposition phase, the body's defense processes can't completely expel the toxins, which have to go somewhere. So they become encased in the connective tissue (mesenchyme), adipose tissue, and throughout the vascular system. Homotoxins that are not expelled from the body are dangerous, and basically need to be deposited and locked into cells and tissues where they can't cause more damage. Research has shown that the increase in obesity rates is a direct result of overexposure to environmental toxins. The body tries to protect itself from damaging toxins by storing them away for a later time when it can properly deal with them, but when it can't, over time, the garbage pile overflows.

The Impregnation Phase

In BioMed, the first three phases are generally naturally reversible. The body is reacting, self-defending, reregulating, and self-healing in a healthy way. Defending comes before healing, healing comes after reregulating and regenerating. However, the following three phases become more complex to treat as damage and degeneration begin to occur to organs and tissues. This fourth phase is called the impregnation phase, whereby the deposited toxins from the third phase start to interfere with enzymatic functions of the cell, like hornets in your car interfere when you are trying to drive. In this fourth stage a process called *loco minoris resistentiae* occurs. Here serious chronic inflammation presents in previously damaged or weakened tissue or organs. Toxins are attracted to and accumulate in tissues and organs that are already damaged, as they have less ability to defend themselves, which is why people who have a past injury will have flare-ups when they get sick or when the barometric pressure drops. When the accumulation of toxins progresses, chronic inflammation ensues. Standard allopathic pain treatment with NSAIDs, cortisone, or opioids basically acts like a stun gun, paralyzing regulatory detoxification processes. Bioregulatory medicine, on the other hand, supports the detoxification process and also attempts to cool inflammation.

Once we get to this fourth phase, chronic conditions start presenting. At this phase the body has to mount a continuous effort in an attempt to restore normal functioning. It is in this phase that some type of intervention is required; the self-healing processes of the body have been exceeded. The record has reached the end and keeps skipping. Without intervention, the body will not be able to regenerate and heal.

Another important element of disease evolution also begins in this fourth phase: Symptoms begin to present in systems unrelated to the original cause. For example, eczemas are often manifestations of lung disorders, whereas neurological manifestations stemming from gastrointestinal disorders show up as multiple sclerosis or myelopathy.[6] And this is the exact moment when allopathic medicine starts to fail when it comes to chronic and degenerative illness. It starts down the wrong trail and treats symptoms, not causes. Eczema—an alarm bell from the lungs—is treated with antibiotics or steroids in allopathic medicine. In contrast, when it comes to skin, bioregulatory medicine starts by looking at the lung or digestive tract, because skin is the first system to compensate for a lung or digestive imbalance. Eczema might be addressed with probiotics, an anti-inflammatory such as fish oil, or various oxygen treatments. Bioregulatory treatments stimulate and support the body to detoxify, regenerate, and self-heal.

The Degeneration Phase

The fifth phase of disease evolution is known as the degeneration phase. In this phase both organ structure and function are increasingly and often irreversibly damaged. Here a continued degenerative alteration of cellular membranes, enzymes, and genetic and organic structures of the cells has occurred. Toxin accumulation continues, adding to the chronic inflammatory response, and the body can't keep up. In this phase it feels like trying to rise to the surface for air when someone is holding your head under water. Loss of energy occurs and organs and tissues cannot repair or regenerate. This phase is where bioregulatory energy medicine treatments (homeopathic, magnetic, oxygen, etc.) have the ability to turn the process around.

The Neoplasm Phase

The final phase of disease evolution is called the neoplasm phase. *Neoplasm* means a new and abnormal growth of tissue in some part of the body, the classic characteristic of cancer. In the neoplasmatic phase, genetic material and metabolic mechanisms are severely damaged. Oxidative free radicals foster further organ dysfunction and tissue degeneration; the bad guys have built their own castles within the walls of the overrun tissues and organs. This is end-stage, chronic, and degenerative illness. This phase is where, in allopathy, we see the most aggressive and toxic treatments, such as high-dose chemotherapy. This phase is where, in bioregulatory medicine, the branches of treatment options grow, extending into the anthroposophical, and diving deeper into energetic, emotional, and spiritual medicine.

Though often presented as bad luck or happenstance by allopathic doctors, we know disease does not come out of nowhere. But because of the nature of allopathic medicine's diagnostics, disease is not detectable until it passes the first three phases. And therefore, a first trip to the doctor to assess symptoms can result in a late-stage diagnosis. The beauty of bioregulatory medicine is that it employs a diagnostic approach that identifies dysregulation *before* it manifests into pathology. Before the castle of health tumbles into the moat. Dysregulation causes a cascade of body-wide events, so next we'll discuss the pinnacle of bioregulatory medicine—its comprehensive body-wide diagnostics. For this discussion, the function of each and every bioregulating system must first be evaluated.

An Introduction to Your Bioregulatory Systems

The human body is a highly complex biophysiological and biochemical network of interconnected and intercommunicating molecules, cells, tissues, and organs. This network includes twelve different bioregulating systems. Therefore, what is called systems biology is the primary scientific backdrop in the bioregulatory medical approach. Systems biology provides a whole-body understanding with a multiscale and multilevel lens. The complexity of a systems-based approach challenges the reductionist/specialist thinking we talked about in chapter 1, and creates the framework for holistic healing.

In humans, homeostasis, is the tendency to resist change in order to maintain a stable, relatively constant internal environment. Typically, maintaining homeostasis involves the action of negative feedback loops that counteract any change to a set point. Negative feedback loops oppose a stimulus or cue. The hallmark of a negative feedback loop is that it counteracts a change, bringing the value of a parameter—such as temperature or blood sugar—back toward a set point. Maintaining homeostasis can be likened to Sir Isaac Newton's third law of motion: For every action, there is an equal and opposite reaction. An example of a feedback loop in the human body is maintenance of body temperature. We'll use temperature as the stimulus for our example. The ideal temperature, or set point, of the human body is 98.6°F, as this is where the thousands of enzymatic systems in the body work most efficiently. Any change to this temperature will be detected by receptors abundant throughout the nervous system, the intestines, the lymphatic system, and the mesenchyme.

The mesenchymal system (also called the interstitium) refers to the spaces between tissues. The mesenchymal system is similar to a wireless network of the body and is critical for homeostatic coordination of cellular communication. The body's billions of receptors are protein molecules that monitor our internal and external environments—similar to a home thermostat or the cruise control system in your car—and convey communication to the temperature regulatory control center in the brain, the hypothalamus. Along with regulating biorhythms, the hypothalamus also regulates many physiologic functions: temperature, thirst, hunger, sleep cycles, blood pressure, heart rate, and the release of hormones including thyroid hormones. This control center then determines the appropriate response and course of action. Is your temperature getting too high? The body will lower it by activating the sweat glands and dilating blood vessels. These commands are considered the output—the energetic instructions—sent from the control center to the regulatory systems in order to illicit a rebalancing reaction.

Clear communication throughout the body is essential; when this communication is disrupted, it's like what happens when all the traffic lights in downtown New York City go out: chaos. There is a highly orchestrated pattern to those traffic lights—they do not change color arbitrarily, rather they are set based on maximizing traffic flow. In the body, communication and regulation are also set based on a formula, flow, or pattern. Each bioregulatory system has its own unique energy flow, feedback loops, and regulation processes to maintain homeostasis. BioMed works by identifying which systems are out of balance and to what extent, and then using natural and noninvasive treatments to repair and regenerate them. Let's look closer at some of our bioregulating systems, the conditions that can affect them, and the difference between how allopathic and bioregulatory medicine assess and treat them.

Cardiovascular System

The heart and circulatory system make up your cardiovascular system. Your heart functions as a pump, or pressure valve, pushing oxygen- and nutrient-containing blood to every organ, tissue, and cell of your body. Blood also removes carbon dioxide and cellular waste products, as does the lymphatic system. Humans carry five pints of blood from the heart to the rest of the body through a complex network of arteries, arterioles, and capillaries. Heart and blood vessel disease—also called heart disease—includes numerous problems, many of which are related to a process called athero-sclerosis. Atherosclerosis is a condition that develops when plaque builds up along arterial walls—like a sink pipe clogged with hair. This buildup narrows the arteries, making it harder for blood to flow through. If a blood clot forms, it can stop the blood flow, causing a heart attack or stroke. Coronary artery disease is the most common type of heart disease in the United States. Currently, heart disease is the leading cause of death for both men and women. About 630,000 Americans die from heart disease annually, accounting for one in every four deaths.

The typical Western medical diagnostic screen for cardiovascular disease is serum cholesterol and triglyceride levels. That's all that allopathic care offers. However, research in the past five years has shown that cholesterol is not, in fact, the best marker to test for heart disease, and that better markers include C-reactive protein and homocysteine. And as we learned in Gary Taube's best-seller *Good Calories, Bad Calories*, the diet-cholesterol-heart-disease myth was largely propelled by makers of statin drugs, and total sales of statins are currently estimated to approach $1 trillion worldwide by 2020. The most commercially successful drug in history, atorvastatin (Lipitor), had sales exceeding $120 billion between 1996 and 2011. To sell more drugs—which is the only allopathic approach to heart disease—we've seen changes to the lab markers for what constitutes both high cholesterol and high blood pressure in the past forty years. In the 1980s, what was considered "high cholesterol" went from 250 total in men down to 200 total for both men and women. More sales of drugs ensued. In the fall of 2017, the American College of Cardiology and the American Heart Association issued a report that said normal blood pressure was considered under 130/80 mmHg, whereas normal had previously been considered under 140/90 mmHg. More sales. But with more drug sales does not come fewer people dying from cardiovascular disease.

In BioMed clinics, every person who walks through the door gets a heart rate variability (HRV) test. This is not a stress test or an echocardiogram, rather it is a noninvasive, efficient diagnostic tool that assesses heartbeats and intervals between heartbeats in a reclined position and a standing position in order to assess the heart's biophysiology and interconnectedness with the autonomic nervous system. The machine also provides a quick and easy assessment of the autonomic nervous system function. Linking the cardiovascular system to the nervous system is critical, as there is an enormous amount of literature showing the links between stress, artery inflammation, and subsequent risk of a heart attack. Primary care physicians will tell their patients to reduce stress, but that's as far as they go. Reduction of stress is important, but what is key is the methods used to control the stress. The HRV test tells the bioregulatory medicine practitioner many things, including circulation analysis and a forecast of the risk for cardiovascular disease.

By identifying cardiovascular dysregulation in the early stages, bioregulatory medicine is able to reverse evolution of the disease using treatment strategies outlined in the next four chapters, which include supplying key spark-plug nutrients such as magnesium that are required by the heart for proper function.

Digestive System

The hollow organs of the digestive system, or the gastrointestinal tract, are the mouth, esophagus, stomach, small intestine, large intestine, and anus. The liver, pancreas, and gallbladder are the solid, accessory organs of the digestive system that have the important job of processing and breaking down food. As a whole, the digestive system converts food into basic nutrients required to feed the entire body—a big job. In the United States, between sixty and seventy million people are affected by digestive diseases, including constipation, diverticulosis, gallstones, GERD, irritable bowel syndrome, celiac disease, ulcerative colitis or Crohn's, different kinds of liver diseases that lead to vitamin K deficiency, fatty liver, portal vein stenosis, cirrhosis, and pancreatic malfunction due to persisting inflammatory processes. Sadly, most people don't know they have a storm brewing in their digestive system until they have pronounced symptoms or dysfunction.

In the allopathic model, the only screening and assessments for digestive health are a few enzymatic tests on an annual blood draw and the required over-age-fifty colonoscopy. This assessment falls short for the adult population and doesn't even touch the pediatric population. Estimates now show that one in eight children have a digestive disorder. Exposing children to blood draws and painful colonoscopies is usually not a parent's first choice. So, sadly, many children live with chronic digestive complaints and are prescribed acid-blocking drugs that deplete them of key nutrients such as vitamin B_{12}, which is required for DNA synthesis, methylation, and genetic health. Bioregulatory medicine, however, offers several noninvasive and pain-free ways to assess digestive health, from stool sample testing to electrodermal acupuncture, thermoregulation assessment to biofeedback, and biocybernetic parasitic to bacterial overgrowth diagnostics. These tests are routine and are part of the standard of care in BioMed clinics. They should be standard in allopathic offices, but sadly many gastroenterologists are not familiar with them; nor do they know how to read the BioMed test results.

Endocrine System

The endocrine system is a collection of glands including but not limited to the hypothalamus, pituitary gland, thyroid, parathyroid, adrenal glands, pancreas, pineal gland, ovaries, and testes. These glands secrete hormones directly into the circulatory system to target organs providing critical biochemical communication and feedback loop coordination within the body. The endocrine system has many functions, including balancing blood sugar, estrogen levels, and metabolism and maintaining stress hormones. That's a lot of work for one system to do, and given our modern diets and lifestyles, it's not able to do it very well. Infertility now affects one in ten women. Endocrine disorders from type 2 diabetes to breast cancer to hypothyroidism affect more than 50 percent of the population. That's a lot of people.

Despite this prevalence, most allopathic primary care providers are not properly assessing patients' hormones. When it comes to blood sugar, for example, most people get a fasting glucose marker run each year—if they are lucky—an HBA1C (a test that gives a three-month average of your blood sugar). People with clear prediabetes are often given no treatment until they have full-blown diabetes, at which point they can be prescribed medications that might include insulin. In general, hormones such as cortisol or estrogen are not part of allopathic prevention screenings. When it comes to hormone imbalance, natural menstrual cycles and menopause are being treated like diseases. Women are placed on birth control pills and hormone replacement therapy (HRT) like they're candy, without baseline assessments to determine hormone levels.

When it comes to prescribing hormones without evaluation, there are two issues. First, the symptoms of estrogen dominance and low estrogen are extremely similar—so a menopausal woman can be placed on estrogen replacement when she already has high estrogen.

Second, why isn't anyone figuring out where hormone symptoms such as PMS are coming from in the first place? Add HRT to estrogen dominance and you have a recipe for estrogen-driven cancers such as breast cancer or ovarian cancer, which now affect one in eight women. The allopathic treatment approach to the endocrine system can be dangerous.

When allopathic physicians run hormone labs, they typically run serum (blood) labs. For many hormones, including estrogen and cortisol, serum testing is not particularly valid. Unfortunately, serum hormone tests do not reflect the full picture of bound versus unbound hormones, nor do they look at DHEA levels, which is one of the precursors to all hormones. DHEA is critical in many disorders and is essential to properly understanding most chronic conditions. It is a disservice to place women on hormone replacements or various fertility treatment programs rather than getting at the root cause of the imbalance, whether it is a gluten sensitivity affecting the thyroid, low progesterone causing infertility, exposure to xenobiotics driving irregular tissue growth in breast, uterus, and ovarian tissue, or a low-fat diet causing the adrenal deficiencies that drive most menopausal symptoms. Western medicine hasn't kept up with advances in diagnostics when it comes to endocrine disorders. BioMed has: Either saliva or a twenty-four-hour urine test is the gold standard for assessing the health of the endocrine system.

Lymphatic System

Considered the unknown or forgotten system, the lymphatic system is a perfect example of just how interconnected each system is. Not only is it part of the circulatory system but it is also a vital part of the immune system. Its interconnective activity is so important. The lymphatic system includes the bone marrow, spleen, tonsils, thymus, lymph nodes, and lymphatic vessels (a network of thin tubes that carry lymph and white blood cells throughout the body). The primary function of the lymphatic system is to transport lymph, a fluid containing infection-fighting white blood cells. If cancer cells break away from a tumor, one of the first places they head is to lymph nodes. Lymphatic vessels branch, like blood vessels, into all the tissues of the body, including the brain, making them the ideal super-highway for metastasizing cancer cells. The lymphatic system also cleanses every cell and organ in the body, providing a pathway for toxins to be removed from the body. When is the last time someone talked to you about your lymphatic system? Probably never, as this is the one system for which allopathic medicine has no specialist.

Yet, every patient with chronic or degenerative disease has a problem with the lymphatic system. Why? Because unlike the cardiovascular system, the lymphatic system has no pump, and it depends on movement from the body for it to circulate. Sadly, our modern lifestyles have most adults sitting at a computer all day and so many—if not most—of us experience lymphatic congestion. Lymphatic congestion can also be caused by injury, surgery, poor diet, emotional/stress states, environmental toxins, hormone imbalances, and normal aging processes. When congestion occurs, these blockages cause a backup in the flow of lymphatic fluid, resulting in swelling or edema in the tissues, called lymphedema. Consequently, toxic waste matter cannot effectively be released from the body, the immune system can't function at optimal performance, and infections, blockages, and acute diseases or chronic diseases, such as cancer, can occur.

The most common complaint in medicine is fatigue. When people feel sluggish, it is often related to their stagnant lymph. Yet the lymphatic system is ignored, and we push through fatigue with coffee, energy drinks, sugar, and alcohol. However, the lymphatic system is a primary focus in BioMed. Tired is not normal, *vital* is. Lymph health is assessed through one or more of at least five different lymphatic testing methods, including electrodermal acupuncture, thermoregulation, iris diagnostics, foot reflexology, and dark-field microscopy. Removing lymphatic congestion is like moving the log out of the flowing river—more nutrients are supplied to cells, toxins are removed, circulation is improved, drainage of excess fluid occurs, collagen formation improves, and immune function increases. Patients wake up, and the fog lifts. Lymphatic treatment technologies such as the Lymphstar or Indiba machines have proven effective for breast health, pain, edema, immune issues, postoperative and injury healing, rejuvenation of the skin, hormone balancing, and to decrease stress. Tired? It's time to find out more about your lymphatic system.

Immune System

The immune system, which is largely made up of lymphatic organs, is a key system when it comes to chronic and degenerative illness. The purpose of the immune system is to keep microorganisms, such as certain bacteria, viruses, and fungi, in balance in the body, and also to destroy any infectious microorganisms that do invade it. The immune system is made up of a complex and vital network of microbes, cells, and organs. There are two arms of the immune system: the innate and the acquired. We are born with what is called innate immunity, which is responsible for our nonspecific defenses. Epithelial surfaces and the skin act like physical barriers to prevent invaders from penetrating our bodies. Acquired immunity is just that: It is obtained from the development of antibodies in response to exposure to an antigen, as from attack from an infectious disease or from the transmission of antibodies from mother to fetus through the placenta.

The innate immune system identifies anything that is foreign (non-self) as a target for an immune response—flu germs, for example. Yet this system has become out of balance in modern times: Over eighty different autoimmune diseases have been identified, and now one in five people have an autoimmune disorder such as celiac disease, lupus, or type 1 diabetes. In autoimmune disease, the body mistakenly attacks itself. Where bioregulatory medicine works to support and restore the function and communication of the immune system by using dozens of different nontoxic and noninvasive treatments, allopathic medicine takes aim at a genetic target and fires at it with immunosuppressive drugs such as steroids. The primary approach of the allopathic medical system is to suppress the systems designed to help us heal. And that is why we don't have cures in the allopathic realm for autoimmune conditions such as multiple sclerosis and rheumatoid arthritis; we have only symptom-suppressing drugs.

When it comes to diagnostics for the immune system, allopathic doctors will run routine CBC tests each year, looking at various white blood cells. That is the extent of their immune assessments. It's like looking at a car and saying it has enough gas without checking the gauge. Yet there are many detectable threats to the immune system—estimates are that up to 90 percent of Americans are deficient in critical immune nutrients, including vitamins D and C, yet these are rarely tested. Bioregulatory medicine places a big focus on immune assessment, restoration, and fortification. Assessments including heavy-metal burden, comprehensive stool tests, cancer screenings, saliva tests, genetic testing of cytokine, interferon and enzymatic detoxification function, lymphocyte profiling, chemosensitivity tests of natural substances, and nutrient testing are standard. If the immune system is depleted, treatments including intravenous vitamins and antioxidants and the powerful, natural immunotherapy, mistletoe, are just a few of the approaches utilized. In contrast, the immunosuppressant drugs used in allopathic medicine reduce the strength of the body's immune system. These drugs are the primary treatment for conditions such as psoriasis, lupus, rheumatoid arthritis, Crohn's disease, multiple sclerosis, and alopecia. In the short term, these drugs have a place in the case of organ transplants, for example, but when it comes to autoimmune conditions, using immunosuppressant drugs confuses and depletes the immune system. The cure comes from correcting the causes of confusion, not simply turning the whole system off. Allopathic medicine is dismissive medicine, medicine that says "let's just lock this process in the basement." The allopathic belief is that you can't cure an autoimmune disease, you just need to try to control the symptoms and delay the inevitable progression until death. Bioregulatory medicines says bring it out of the locked basement, nurture it, and get it back on its feet.

Musculoskeletal System

The musculoskeletal system is the body's interconnected system of nerves, muscles, and bones. Anatomy is the study of body-part structure, while physiology studies the function of body parts. One of the guiding principles in both anatomy and physiology is called the principle of complementarity, which states that function is dependent on structure, and that the form of a structure relates to its function. Structure equals function. When there is no pain, it's easy to take our bones and muscles for granted. The structure of the musculoskeletal system allows painless movement and function to happen. Skeletal muscles move the 206 bones in the adult body. Smooth muscles are found within the organs, and they propel food down the esophagus to the stomach, through the intestines, and out the other end. Our heart is a smooth muscle. The bones are also very active—even when not in motion. The skeletal system is responsible for blood cell production, calcium storage, and endocrine regulation. The bone marrow inside of all the bones in the human skeletal system contains stem cells. These stem cells develop into the red blood cells that carry oxygen through the body, the white blood cells that fight infections, and the platelets that help with blood clotting. The skeletal system is also part of the immune system, and the muscular system is part of the digestive system.

So, when this system is dysregulated, function decreases. Decreased function in the musculoskeletal system often presents as pain. Today, more than one hundred million Americans suffer from chronic pain—more than three times as many people as have diabetes. Allopathic medicine's answer: surgery, opioid drugs, and nonsteroidal anti-inflammatories. We've already discussed the opioid crisis in the United States, and many allopathic doctors have been cited for malpractice for overprescribing opioids. Drugs are *not* the answer. In contrast, both osteopathic and chiropractic medicines and massage therapy—all modalities employed by BioMed—have a special focus on the musculoskeletal system. These modalities provide drug-free, noninvasive manual therapies that aim to improve health across all body systems by manipulating and strengthening the musculoskeletal framework—the joints, muscles, and spine. Conditions including acid reflux, tendinitis, carpal tunnel syndrome, osteoarthritis, rheumatoid arthritis, and fibromyalgia are related to this system. By addressing the body's structure, function follows suit.

Nervous System

The nervous system is a highly complex network of nerves and cells that carries messages to and from the brain and spinal cord to various parts of the body. The central nervous system is made up of the brain and spinal cord, and the peripheral nervous system is made up of the somatic and the autonomic nervous systems. The somatic nervous system consists of peripheral nerve fibers that pick up sensory information, or sensations, from the peripheral or distant organs (such as the arms and legs) and carry them to the central nervous system. There are three parts to the autonomic nervous system: the sympathetic nervous system (regulating fight or flight), the parasympathetic nervous system (regulating rest and digest), and the enteric nervous system. The autonomic nervous system controls the nerves of the inner organs, over which humans have no conscious control, including heartbeat, digestion, and breathing. Our nervous system is influenced by our environment and adjusts our internal environment accordingly. A major function of the nervous system—along with the endocrine system—is to control homeostasis.

Neurological disorders are diseases of the brain and spine and the nerves that connect them. There are more than six hundred diseases of the nervous system, such as brain tumors, epilepsy, ALS, Alzheimer's disease, and Parkinson's disease. Yet the function of the nervous system is not assessed from a prevention standpoint in allopathic medicine. Not at all. Meanwhile, stress, poor diet, nutrient depletions (B vitamins and DHA fatty acid are critical for brain health), lack of exercise, and environmental toxins wreak havoc on the health of the nervous system. Bioregulatory medicine takes the health of the nervous system into account when assessing chronic and degenerative diseases and also performance. Balance between the sympathetic and parasympathetic nervous systems is essential, and this is often achieved using BioMed therapies, including neurofeedback, a state-of-the-art, noninvasive, drugless method for teaching the brain to function in a more balanced and healthful way. Usually considered simple and pleasant, neurofeedback can help shift the way the brain produces and distributes its electrical energy. We will go much deeper into this and other elements of the neurological system in chapter 7, but for now it's important to understand that the nervous system has cross talk and interaction with internal and external environments, and keeping it healthy is a critical piece of the disease-prevention puzzle. BioMed clinics are where to go for comprehensive prevention diagnostic testing—the days of a CBC and a basic physical exam have expired.

Urinary System

The urinary system consists of all the organs involved in the formation and release of urine. It includes the kidneys, ureters, bladder, and urethra. The urinary system also helps us regulate the amount of glucose, salts, and water in the blood. The kidneys—considered the powerhouse of the body in TCM and bioregulatory medicine—filter the blood to remove wastes and produce urine. They also maintain the body's acid-base balance by reabsorbing bicarbonate from urine or excreting hydrogen ions into urine. Blood is normally slightly basic, with a normal pH range of 7.35 to 7.45, and this is maintained largely by the urinary system. Allopathic medicine does sometimes screen for acid-alkaline balance and also looks at a few different serum kidney markers, especially in diabetic patients. BioMed assesses all the same diagnostic markers that allopathic medicine does, but uses many more tests for every system. For urinary system health, testing includes regulation thermography, urine tests, and Zyto scans. Proper acid-alkaline balance determines the body's regulatory mechanisms and is specifically addressed in bioregulatory medicine. The urinary system plays a critical role in both detoxification and the important homeostatic process of maintaining blood pH. We will learn more about protein and pH in chapter 5, but the key is that the kidneys play a huge role in our health and vitality.

Respiratory System

The human respiratory system is a series of organs responsible for taking in oxygen and expelling carbon dioxide. The primary organs of the respiratory system are the lungs, which carry out this gas exchange as we breathe. The breathing process is aided by a large dome-shaped muscle under the lungs called the diaphragm. Mucus is produced by cells in the trachea and bronchial tubes, intended to stop dust, bacteria, viruses, and allergy-causing substances from entering the lungs. Lung cancer is currently one of the most common types of cancers worldwide and affects more nonsmokers every year. Rates of allergies, asthma, and chronic obstructive pulmonary disease (COPD) have surged in the past fifty years as well. As we know, in order to stay alive, the human body requires oxygen, nutrients, and water. Oxygen, devoid of toxic pollutants, is a very powerful health-giving substance. For both the treatment of disease and for improving performance in athletes, bioregulatory medicine places a large focus on the importance of oxygen. Nontoxic, noninvasive treatments, including ozone therapy and exercise with oxygen therapy, are highly effective for improving the health of the respiratory system.

Ozone therapy has been utilized and studied for more than a century. Its benefits are proven, consistent, safe, and it has minimal and preventable side effects. Medical ozone is used to disinfect and treat disease. Ozone therapy inactivates bacteria, viruses, fungi, yeasts, and protozoa while activating the immune system—a great therapy to counteract today's toxic indoor and outdoor environments. Various ozone treatments have also been found to be highly effective in addressing Lyme disease, an increasingly common chronic bacterial infection for which allopathic medicine has a single treatment: antibiotics. Sufferers of Lyme's disease can spend decades—if not their entire life—experiencing dysregulation of the respiratory, immune, neurological, digestive, and other systems. Allopathic medicine has nothing to offer to address these dysregulations aside from anti-inflammatories and antidepressants. BioMed, on the other hand, uses treatments such as hydrotherapy, neurofeedback, intravenous vitamin C, probiotics, energy therapy, and especially oxygen therapies to restore quality of life for these patients.

Another effective oxygen treatment involves the practice of breathing a high flow rate of "oxygen-enriched air" (90 percent and above) while exercising. This treatment has been shown to provide dramatic health benefits and prevent cancer, macular degeneration, cataracts, diabetes, chronic fatigue, and fibromyalgia. Exercise with Oxygen Training, or EWOT, has been used by professional sports teams for years; it involves simply breathing high levels of oxygen while exercising. The effects cause an increase in the oxygen-carrying capability of the red blood cells, the blood plasma, and the fluid portion of the blood. This increases performance and lung health, and has been found to be an effective cancer therapy as cancer cells thrive in low-oxygen environments but do poorly when a high level of oxygen is present.

For all of these systems (with the exception of the lymphatic), there is a specialist in allopathic medicine who devotes their career to that one system alone. For heart issues we go to the cardiologist, a rheumatologist diagnoses and treats musculoskeletal and autoimmune diseases, urologists treat conditions that affect the urinary system and the male reproductive system, while endocrinologists treat the female reproductive system and other hormone imbalances. Each specialist has his or her own set of pharmaceutical and surgical protocols. But there should be only one specialization in medicine: the patient. The patterns and connections between systems are critical, including the hypothalamic-pituitary-adrenal (HPA) axis and the psycho-neuro-endocrine-immune (PNEI) system (which we cover in more detail in forthcoming chapters). The human body is complex, and it needs a medical model that understands this complexity. Now that we have had a little introduction into some of the systems and their associated dysregulations, the next four chapters will go deep into four core treatment focuses of BioMed: detoxification and therapeutic drainage, nutrition, nervous system calibration (including mental and emotional components), and oral health.

CHAPTER FOUR

Detoxification
Homotoxicology and Biotherapeutic Drainage

All things are poison and nothing is without poison, only the dose permits something not to be poisonous.

—PARACELSUS

Diseases are the expression of biological purposeful defense mechanisms against endogenic and exogenic homotoxins, or the expression of the organism's effort to compensate for toxic damages it has sustained.

—DR. H. H. RECKEWEG, MD

U p until around three hundred years ago, when the fossil-fueled motors of the Industrial Revolution started spinning, the only poisonous materials humans had ever encountered were organic substances of animal, plant, mineral, metal, viral, or microbial origin: a shiny leaf, a venomous snake, a drink from a dirty pond. As a species, we've had a lot of time to adapt to these biotoxins, or poisonous substances produced by living organisms (such as red tide), as well as the ninety or so naturally occurring yet toxic-to-human elements such as plutonium. For the past six million years, humans have coevolved with—and been consumers of—plants, animals, minerals, metals, and microbes. In fact, as many as 145 human genes were transferred from viruses, bacteria, archaea, fungi, and animals.[1] Not only do our bodies react to the biorhythms of the planet, but humans are also part of the planet.

For example, 18 percent of our body mass is carbon. In our bodies, the ratio between resident microbes and human cells is estimated between 1:1 and 10:1, and approximately 1 percent of our genome comes from plants that contain naturally occurring toxic, repellent, and even pharmacodynamic compounds designed to counter attacks from us and other herbivores. Through the millennia, the various regulatory systems in our bodies—especially our immune systems—evolved to recognize and respond to these naturally occurring biotoxins and elements identified on the periodic table. We have acquired genetically adapted thresholds of how many of them our systems can handle before we get sick or die. It is the dose and duration of exposure that makes a substance poisonous, or, in some cases, medicinal.

The term *hormesis* is the definition of a biological dose effect. This process is a phenomenon whereby a beneficial effect can result from low-dose exposures to an agent that is toxic or lethal at higher doses. For example, when Romeo slugged a vial of the purple-flowered monkshood in Shakespeare's *Romeo and Juliet*, it killed him. But, when ingested at a specific homeopathic dose, *Aconitum napellus*, the same plant, exerts immune-boosting effects. This hormetic concept of dose-makes-the-poison is why today allopathic medicine is using oncolytic viruses—live viruses such as the poliovirus—to try to kill cancer. It appears that many biotoxic agents have antitumor, immunomodulatory, and apoptotic effects.[2] The dose response is the fine line between therapeutic and detrimental; it's the threshold between where dose and duration moves from what we can tolerate to what we cannot, to which symptoms we have and which we don't. Even water can be fatal if we drink too much at once. Yet thresholds are highly individual. Variations in anatomy, body composition, enzyme patterns, endocrine activities, excretion patterns, genetics, basal metabolism, bacterial flora, nutrient absorption and utilization, constitution, miasm, and lifestyle tolerances can all impact our response to a substance. Two people can drink the same amount of alcohol at a dinner party yet have two very different responses.

To avoid extinction, our bodies developed highly complex coping mechanisms to deal with harmful biotoxins and elements such as hemlock and cinnabar. These mechanisms, called hormetic pathways or stress response pathways, involve adaptive changes in cells and molecules that regulate and encourage cytoprotection, a process where various proteins in our bodies provide and activate cellular protection against harmful agents, much like, if your body were a car, it has airbags and other automobile safety features. One of these protective hormetic stress resistance proteins is the inflammation and immune activator NF-κB, which acts like an emergency first responder, and is involved with communicating and activating specific responses to external stimuli such as stress, injury, poisonous plant ingestion, pathogenic bacteria, or virus. NF-κB is active and protective in the second phase of disease evolution, the reaction phase, as well.

Another example of our body's inherent protective responses are the antioxidant enzymes superoxide dismutase, glutathione peroxidase, and catalase. Each cell makes these to protect itself from the damaging effects of free radicals, including reactive oxygen species (ROS). ROS is a normal product of cellular metabolism—like exhaust from a car. ROS is an internal, or endogenous, toxin or waste product produced from normal metabolic activities such as breathing, exercising, and digesting. However, ROS and all other free radicals cause damage to healthy cells by stealing their electrons. Other endogenous free radicals include carbon dioxide, urea, and lactic acid. Our bodies churn out these oxidative-stress–inducing toxins by the second, and, when in balance, our bodies are well equipped to neutralize them with antioxidant enzymes. But every bioregulating system has its threshold and can only handle so much before response pathways become blocked, overloaded, dysregulated, and then fail. When there is an overaccumulation of internal or external toxins, this antioxidant enzyme system becomes overwhelmed and dysregulated.

Fast-forward through human evolution to three hundred years ago, into the smokestacked high-rises of modern life. During the last few hundred years the most common causes of death have changed from communicable to noncommunicable, from acute to chronic.

The biggest threats to human mortality morphed from acute and biotoxic in origin (i.e., eat a poisonous mushroom and die) to chronic, lingering disease states, such as a ten-year cancer battle. The precipitating factor in this shift is the almost incomprehensive deluge of eighty thousand new types of toxins that have entered the planet's biosphere: xenobiotics (also referred to as homotoxins in bioregulatory medicine) are synthetic, man-made, chemical toxins created by artificial processes. These toxins are foreign both to human biological systems and to the systems of our planet. Since the Industrial Revolution, we've swiftly converted to a lifestyle dominated by machine manufacturing, petrochemically derived products, fossil-fueled transportation, corporate agriculture, and fabricated pharmaceuticals. In a very, very short amount of time, the chemical industry learned how to convert naturally occurring materials such as oil, natural gas, air, water, metals, and minerals into inorganic chemicals used for consumer and industrial products that are not, in many cases, biodegradable. Nonbiodegradable substances are those that cannot be transformed into a harmless natural state by bacterial action. Instead, they persist (e.g., plastics). But three hundred years, in the span of human existence, is akin to one letter in a five-hundred-page novel, or a finger snap in a twenty-four-hour day. Before that time there were no plastics, no televisions, no exhaust fumes, no vaccinations, no fluoride, no synthetic foods, no synthetic fibers, no fragranced laundry detergent, no BPA, no flame-retardant-coated couches, no endocrine-disrupting body care products, no genetically altered foods, no toxic cleaning products, no antibiotics, no synthetic hormones, no electricity, no airplanes, no pesticides, no wireless networks, no Tylenol, no dioxins, no preservatives. This list of xenobiotics could go on for five hundred more pages. And odds are, you've been exposed to many of them. With the advent of industry, which relies heavily on petroleum for energy, humans have become barraged with a whole new type of foreign xenobiotics.

The list of what we (and our immune and antioxidant systems) were exposed to prior to the advent of industry included only nat-urally occurring biotoxins and elements. *Naturally occurring* means from a living organism or an element that has a molecular structure identified on the periodic table (or a combination thereof). Organic substances also always contain a carbon. Carbon is the foundation of life, produced by or derived from all living—biological—organisms. In fact, all living organisms are built of carbon compounds and all living organisms, including people, require carbon in order to live, grow, and reproduce. In the previous chapter we discussed some of the biocycles of the planet, and the carbon cycle is one of them. The carbon cycle is a biogeochemical cycle whereby carbon is rotated among plants, people, oceans, the atmosphere, ecosystems, and geosphere. Plants, for example, absorb carbon dioxide from the atmosphere to facilitate glucose in creating photosynthesis, which in turn provides fuel for the plant cells to operate. Glucose is a molecule made up of carbon, hydrogen, and oxygen. In the natural world, everywhere you look there is carbon.

However, *altered* forms of carbon can exert highly xenotoxic effects. Polycyclic aromatic hydrocarbons (PAHs), for example, are chemicals released when organic materials such as coal, petroleum, or wood are burned in cars, airplanes, homes, and machines. PAHs are also used in pharmaceuticals, agricultural products, synthetic fibers, detergents, and more. In addition to heating the planet at an alarming rate, PAHs can cause carcinogenic and mutagenic effects and are potent immunosuppressants.[3] Certain PAHs, like benzo[a] pyrene, found in diesel exhaust, are well-known carcinogens, mutagens, and teratogens posing serious threats to human health and well-being. And these PAHs are in many products of daily living. Decreasing, increasing, or altering natural elements, such as carbon, is where we are getting ourselves into deep toxic trouble and is the primary cause of chronic illness.

The nearly one hundred thousand new xenobiotics approved for use in our environment come from many different sources, including landfills, incinerators, factories, electromagnetic smog, chemical pollution, emissions, food production, and pharmaceuticals. In the air, soil, and water, xenobiotics are everywhere. In just a morning routine, we can be exposed to over one hundred different synthetic toxic compounds, from soap ingredients to fluoride in shower water, to perfumes, clothing dyes, dioxins in coffee filters, off-gases from new construction materials, preservatives and additives in foods, engine exhaust during a commute, electromagnetic fields from our cell phones—the list is exhausting and endless in modern times. By the time we get to work, most of us have had a xenobiotic-infused morning. Today, 99 percent of everything we touch—with the exception of each other, our pets, and the earth's natural dirt—has synthetic compounds involved with its production. As evidenced by the alarming increase in disease rates, our bodies are not responding well.

What's horrifying is that less than 5 percent of these toxins have been studied for safety, and none for their synergistic effects—or how they interact with each other. Vinegar is safe and baking soda is safe, but combine the two like we did in eighth-grade chemistry class and you get a volcano. We don't know for sure what a combination of, say, the butylated hydroxytoluene in breakfast cereal and the talc in statin medications is doing. But we do know one thing: There is a huge amount of untested chemicals in our world, and our tolerance thresholds are clearly getting pushed over the edge. Sadly, we've let the wolf watch the sheep when it comes to chemical safety, as our current legislature allows the chemical industry to essentially police themselves. And it's not too surprising how badly it's being handled. There's far too much money to be made to be slowed down by safety issues. In 2016, the global chemical industry's revenue stood at US$5.2 trillion.

While our bioregulating systems are trying to keep pace with a barrage of synthetic external toxins, we are also faced with a new breed of internal toxins. With the addition of synthetic foods, chemical pesticides, and increased sugar, hormones, and antibiotics into our diets, modern humans are now plagued with dysbiotic gastrointestinal tracts. Microbial imbalances allow the overgrowth of pathological bacteria, yeasts, and fungi, which then release toxic gases such as ammonia and acetaldehyde into our digestive systems. Once absorbed, these toxins cause significant disruption of body functions. In fact, gut-derived microbial toxins have been implicated in a wide variety of diseases, including digestive tract cancers, liver disease, Crohn's disease, ulcerative colitis, thyroid disease, lupus, allergies, pancreatitis, asthma, and immune disorders. These toxins are a whole new ball game for our physiology. Considering that half of all Americans have a chronic or degenerative illness, we have to start paying attention to the role these new toxins might be playing in our demise. The problem is, symptoms often sneak in slowly, starting as fatigue and brain fog. They also manifest psychologically—anger, depression, and anxiety can be signs of deep toxicity. These are symptoms we often brush off or mask with lattes and Lexapro. Consider a few of the other signs of toxin overload:

- Frequent, unexplained headaches and back, neck, and joint pain, or arthritis
- Chronic respiratory problems, allergies, or asthma
- Abnormal body odor, bad breath, or coated tongue
- Food allergies, poor digestion, chronic constipation with intestinal bloating or gas
- Brittle nails and hair, psoriasis, adult acne
- Unexplained weight gain or inability to lose weight
- Chronic insomnia
- Unusually poor memory, depressed mood, irritability, and other neurological symptoms including mental confusion, mental illness
- Tingling in hands and feet or abnormal nerve reflexes
- Chronic fatigue, slow starter in the morning
- Problems digesting fatty/creamy/oily foods, and they can make you feel unwell or even nauseous
- Elevated cholesterol, uric acid, or triglycerides
- Environmental sensitivities, especially to odors such as perfume
- Intolerance to alcohol

Back in the 1960s, Rachel Carson's eye-opening masterpiece *Silent Spring* warned the public about the dangers of xenobiotics. Her book explained that toxin exposure levels could not be controlled, and that scientists could not accurately predict the long-term effects of xenobiotic bioaccumulation in our cells nor quantify the impact of chemical mixtures on human health. She was right. We now know that toxin exposures persist through the generations. Just consider what happened with the DES babies. DES (diethylstilbestrol) is a man-made, synthetic form of estrogen prescribed between 1938 and 1971 to pregnant women at risk of miscarriages or premature deliveries. Years later, their daughters and sons and even *their* offspring experience reproductive tract malformations, decreased fertility, and increased risk of endocrine cancers including ovarian and prostate. Despite warnings from Carson and scores of others, environmental pollution and the various forms of homotoxicity have skyrocketed in last couple of decades. Messing with biorhythms and naturally occurring elements has got us swimming in a very scary, dysregulated toxic soup. There is no denying that disease symptoms are the body's inherent response to expelling the massive amounts of toxins that our regulating systems are being exposed to. Why else are we so sick? It is time for the suppression of authentic medicine to end so that people can start living healthy and vital lives. Every year an estimated two thousand new chemicals are introduced for use in everyday items such as food, personal care products, prescription drugs, household cleaners, and lawn care products. And we are getting sicker and sicker.

Most likely, you have no idea how toxic you are. When the Environmental Protection Agency started the National Human Adipose Tissue Survey back in the 1970s, they were curious about the levels of xenobiotics present in human fat cells. Not surprisingly, five highly toxic chemicals including two known carcinogens, benzene and dioxins, were found in 100 percent of all samples. Today, anywhere from fifteen to five hundred synthetic chemicals can be found in measurable quantities in the body fat of every single living human—chemicals such as pesticides, plastics, phthalates, pharmaceuticals, and POPs, or persistent organic pollutants. These chemicals are even found in newborn babies—passed from mom through the placenta. The toxins are highly unstable, and once in the body via ingestion, inhalation, injection, or absorption, they wreak all kinds of havoc. Xenobiotics have detrimental effects on cell structure and function—they cause DNA damage and inflammation, suppress immune function, alter metabolism, disrupt the endocrine system, and cause direct tissue damage.

Toxins are tiny atom bombs blowing holes in homeostasis and are the leading cause of systemic dysregulation. And while we often can't see the effects on the outside, on the inside every single one of our bioregulatory systems is hard at work trying to identify, neutralize, and excrete these foreign synthetic toxins. And they're having a heck of a time trying to keep up.

The Ticking Clock of Toxins in the Body

When the body is exposed to any type of toxin, there are hundreds—if not thousands—of metabolic reactions that take place throughout every single bioregulatory system to help the body return to homeostasis. Toxins can be fatal, depending on dose and duration, so all hands are on deck. There are essentially three steps a bioregulated body uses to appropriately respond to any type of toxin, whether organic or synthetic: recognize, metabolize, and eliminate. This process is a whole-body response that includes our immune, detoxification, lymphatic, hepatic, digestive, and cardio-vascular systems, and more. When any one of these bioregulatory systems is out of balance, snafus in the toxin removal process occur, leading to toxin overaccumulation—and ultimately chronic illness via the six stages of disease development we discussed in chapter 3. The problem is, the rate of xenobiotic exposure has escalated extremely quickly, and our bodies just haven't had time to evolve adaptive mechanisms to respond to all these new chemicals. It's hard to drink from a fire hose.

The first step in toxin recognition is where the immune system has intimate involvement. The major function of the immune system is to protect us from foreign substances—biotoxins and both natural and synthetic elements. Protection is achieved by knowing what elements of the body are "self" and then responding to whatever substances are "nonself." But the key is *recognition*, and our immune systems are now faced with tens of thousands of new xenobiotics that they've never seen or developed antibodies for. A healthy immune system can quickly flag and tag nonself substances, such as *Giardia*, for example. Once something is flagged as foreign the immune system either destroys or neutralizes the substance, which is then further biotransformed by the liver before elimination. The liver is the body's filtration system, and it fulfills many vital tasks—including digestive and hormonal ones—and is responsible for the proper functioning of humans in general, which is why it has such incredible regeneration ability.

Within liver cells, sophisticated processes break down, or metabolize, toxic substances. These same mechanisms are also currently faced with a myriad of new nonself compounds. Like a hamster on a wheel, our livers can have a difficult time making any progress, which leads to dysregulation. Every drug we take, every artificial chemical, pesticide, preservative, or hormone, is metabolized inside our liver cells. The way a toxin is metabolized depends on its size, shape, and solubility, which means whether a substance will dissolve in either water or fat. For example, if you try to mix butter and water, the butter floats on top of the water, which means it's fat-soluble. Salt, on the other hand, will dissolve in water because it's water-soluble. There are fat-soluble toxins and water-soluble toxins. Fat-soluble toxins are harder for the body to excrete whereas water-soluble toxins can be quickly eliminated from the body in urine. It should come as no surprise that the majority of xenobiotics are fat-soluble, making them even more persistent in the body. Think if it like islands of floating plastic inside the oceans of our bodies.

The liver has two primary detoxification pathways designed to convert fat-soluble chemicals into water-soluble chemicals for excretion from the body. These are called the Phase I and Phase II detoxification pathways. Phase I detoxification uses cytochrome P450 enzymes. Phase II detoxification, also called the conjugation pathway, involves liver cells adding another substance, such as cysteine or sulfur, to a toxin rendering it less harmful. Both Phase I and Phase II detoxification are regulated by our genes, use a large amount of antioxidants, and have nutrient requirements in order to function. If you have a single nucleotide polymorphism (SNP) in your various P450 enzymes, then detoxification pathways and processes can be impaired. SNPs are like a hiccup in genetic function. For example, almost 25 percent of all drugs are metabolized by the CYP2D6 protein, including beta-blockers and antidepressants. If a person has a SNP to this gene, then their metabolism of many synthetic drugs will be compromised. What's more, both Phase I and Phase II detoxification have nutrient requirements in order to function, such as vitamin C and magnesium, and over 60 percent of the American adult population is depleted in these nutrients.[4] There are many factors that can impair toxin metabolism. An impaired metabolism becomes a situation where the trash keeps piling up but the dump is always closed.

Today there are many synthetic toxic compounds that the body has difficulty metabolizing and eliminating due to a lack of specific enzymes that we haven't had time to develop yet. Three hundred years is just not enough time to adapt to eighty thousand new chemicals—three hundred thousand years probably wouldn't be enough either. Regardless, the dangerous toxins that are not metabolized can't be left bouncing around causing damage—so the body encases them in adipose (fat) tissue and sends them, stomping their feet, into "time out" in the extracellular matrix, tissues, or organs. This process is the third phase of disease development. Fat-soluble toxins such as heavy metals, including mercury from fish or dental fillings, lead, aluminum, and also synthetic organic molecules such as organophosphates, dioxins, herbicides, colorings, and preservatives, all get deposited within various specific tissues, organs, or connective tissues (the matrix). Research has shown elevated levels of aluminum in the brains of Alzheimer's patients, and elevated levels of lead have been found in the baby teeth of children who are on the autism spectrum. Obesity is the ultimate expression of toxicity—we create fat in order to store toxins. In fact, the commonly held causes of obesity—overeating and inactivity—do not completely explain the current obesity epidemic; research is now pointing at *obesogens*, the term used for the foreign fat-soluble chemical compounds that dysregulate lipid metabolism, as a leading cause of obesity.[5] Atrazine, the second most commonly used herbicide in the United States, is classified as an obesogen and is found on nonorganic corn, sugarcane, and wheat crops. These foreign synthetic chemicals are snarling the hairs of our health, and our waistlines are showing it.

But let's return to the unmetabolized toxins. These are deposited layer by layer inside the cells and tissues of our milieu, like boxes in a garage. The oldest toxins are embedded the deepest. Year by year they get pushed further and further back. These deep toxins cannot be eliminated until the newer ones are removed first—the boxes in front have to be cleared out before we can get to older boxes. The problem is, in modern times, xenobiotic exposure is unrelenting. Unwanted boxes keep coming and the older ones get pushed deeper into the corners. And the more toxins that are stored, the more dysfunction and degeneration specific tissues and organs experience. How can you park the car in the garage if it's full of boxes? You can't, and cells and tissues cannot function properly with toxins in their space either. A toxic tissue, organ, or connective tissue matrix will manifest progressively into serious symptoms ranging from inflammation, cysts, gout, and rheumatism to atherosclerosis, tumors, and cancer. In this way overexposure to toxins, without proper detoxification, leads us into the later, harder-to-treat phases of disease evolution.

In the case of an acute toxic exposure, such as pesticide poisoning or chemotherapy, some of the toxins are stored temporarily and then released at a rate that allows the detoxification organs to keep up. This slow release reduces immediate stress and genotoxic effects on the liver and kidneys especially. The term *late effects* refers to side effects that can occur in some people months or years after cytotoxic drug treatments. Cytotoxic drugs contain chemicals that are toxic to cells and are used to treat cancer, rheumatoid arthritis, and multiple sclerosis. Late-effect symptoms can include fatigue, difficulty with focused thinking, early menopause, heart problems, reduced lung capacity, kidney and urinary problems, nerve problems such as numbness and tingling, and/or bone and joint problems. The long-term outcome of acute or long-term heavy chemical exposure is reversible in some cases and irreversible in others. Reversability depends on the combination of dose, duration, genetic predisposition, and presences of nutrient cofactors required for toxin metabolism. For example, over one third of war veterans exposed to highly toxic agents including organophosphates, carbamates, cyclosarin nerve agents, and pyridostigmine bromide medications experience long-term fatigue, headaches, cognitive dysfunction, depression, fibromyalgia, brain cancer, and respiratory, gastrointestinal, and dermatologic complaints.[6] There is no doubt exposure to toxins causes health issues.

Humans have three inherent mechanisms for the elimination of toxins—temperature (fever), inflammation, and discharge. It is now commonly agreed that *all* chronic and degenerative disease is a result of inflammation. Recall that one of our hormetic response pathways is the activation of NF-κB, which is the mother molecule that actives the inflammatory response. Inflammation is the body's attempt to surround the toxin while the immune system destroys it and the blood carries it away. Fevers permit increased circulation and also have a natural pathogen-killing ability. Fever and inflammation help move along the toxin elimination process. Toxins move from inside the body to outside the body via the emunctory tissues and organs, a process called discharge. The five primary physical emunctories are the skin, gastrointestinal tract (intestines), lung, kidney, and bladder. The central nervous system, which houses many emotions, is also recognized as having emunctory functions. These organs and systems move toxins out of the body in the form of discharges, including urine, feces, vomit, mucus, and sweat. The emunctories are like plumbing in your house, a network of pipes that carry toxic discharges from the inside out. By definition, the liver, stomach, blood, lymph, and pancreas are not tissues that permit removal of wastes to the exterior of the body, but they do perform many essential functions in the detoxification process, which is another reason we need to see the regulatory systems of the body as a whole system, working in concert, not as solo artists.

When our emunctories are working properly, then toxins are removed from the body with little aggravation. When they are not, symptoms will arise in response to healing. What's known as a *healing crisis* can happen when the emunctories are not physiolog-ically functioning normally. That is to say, the body has reached a state where it is incapable of adequately removing all the met-abolically produced endogenous wastes and the accumulated exogenous wastes—the garage is overflowing with boxes and there is no room for more, and some boxes spill into the driveway, getting wet and damaged. Add our highly xenotoxic environments to the conventional medical approach of suppressing illness, and the high emotional stress that is a signature of modern life, and we can see how our regulatory systems can no longer function properly to defend us from toxin overload.

Toxins: The Root Cause of Common Chronic and Degenerative Disease

Xenobiotics specifically target the immune, neurological, and endo-crine systems, explaining the enormous array of common health problems caused directly or indirectly by synthetic toxin overload. Over time, multiple invisible exposures—the morning doughnut, the red nail polish, the dry cleaning—start to build up. Fat-soluble chemicals, such as pesticides and food additives, not only encourage the production of fat to help metabolize and encapsulate them, but also have binding affinity to fatty tissues in, for example, the breast and the brain. In these fatty parts of the body, hard-to-remove toxins accumulate, partially explaining the rampant prevalence of cancers and degenerative diseases in these tissues. Breast cancer is the most common cancer today, affecting one in eight women. The near-three-hundred-page 2012 World Health Organization and International Programme on Chemical Safety document *The Harmonization Project Document #10* should be read by all allopathic doctors who insist we don't know the cause of modern chronic and degenerative illness—especially allergic, autoimmune, neurological, and endocrine disorders. *Document #10* lists twenty "category 1" diseases and disorders that have immunotoxicity as the precipitating factor in their development. *Immunotoxicity* is defined as "adverse effects on the functioning of the immune system as a result of exposure to chemical substances." These include ear infections, autoimmune diseases, asthma, childhood leukemia, multiple sclerosis, rheumatoid arthritis, sarcoidosis, Sjogren's syndrome, and type 1 diabetes. Yes, inner ear infections in children can be caused by toxins.

Because the immune system is the first responder to toxic invasion, it is a highly toxicological target, as it's a fully dispersed bioregulatory system, represented in most tissues, organs, and peripheral sites including the respiratory, dermal, gastrointestinal, neurological, cardiovascular, reproductive, hepatic, and endocrine systems. Whatever way a toxin enters the body, the immune system is the front line of defense to recognize and respond to it. Our immune systems are very busy these days, and unfortunately this bioregulatory system is taking the hardest hit, resulting in immunotoxicity-related diseases such as allergies and autoimmune diseases. Synthetic toxins do all sorts of nasty things to our immune systems: They decrease levels of T cells and lower natural killer cell activity, they depress levels of immunoglobins (antibodies) that attach to xenobiotics, and they assist in destroying the antibodies.

The Epidemic of Autoimmune Disease

Alongside obesity, the autoimmune disease epidemic is a significant consequence of how toxic our environments have become. Rates of autoimmune disease have skyrocketed in the past thirty years; approximately fifty million Americans, 20 percent of the population—or one in five people—suffer from an autoimmune disease. This is absolutely not normal, nor should it be considered the new normal! Briefly, autoimmune disease occurs when the immune system makes an antibody to counteract a toxin, which, in its wake, attacks the tissue it is bound to or stored in. This happens to the thyroid in Hashimoto's thyroiditis and the myelin sheath that surrounds nerve cells in the case of multiple sclerosis. In autoimmune diseases we see elevated antibody levels of certain tissues, including antithyroid antibodies, antimyelin antibodies, and anti-smooth-muscle antibodies. This process is like the police trying to shoot holes in the tires to stop the car of a fugitive. Sadly, in the case of autoimmune conditions, the immune system hits healthy tissue in the crossfire.

Toxins and Cancer

Cancers have clear associations with environmental chemicals. Many xenobiotics have been identified as also genotoxic—including synthetic antibacterial, antiviral, antimalarial, and antifungal drugs. (This is ironic because these are all drugs designed to suppress the body's inherent responses to naturally occurring biotoxic agents.) In addition to pharmaceuticals, higher levels of PCBs, hexachloro-cyclohexane (lice shampoo), and other chemicals have been found in the adipose tissue of breast cancer patients as compared with control groups. In kids, 2,4-D, a common household weed killer (found in Monsanto's Roundup and Ortho's Weed B Gone) is associated with soft tissue carcinomas. No-pest strips and flea collars are associated with leukemia. Reduction in natural killer cell activity that is signature to toxin exposure has been shown to correlate with increased susceptibility to sarcomas and melanomas. Both the skin and the lungs act as barriers between us and the environment, and so they are often directly exposed to environmental toxins. It's not surprising that skin and lung cancers also happen to be two of the most common types of cancer worldwide.

Toxins and Neurological Disease

Neurological diseases, too, are correlated with toxicity; researchers at the Centers for Disease Control and Prevention (CDC) found that between 1999 and 2014 the rate of death from Alzheimer's disease increased by more than 50 percent.[7] Neurotoxins, an extensive class of exogenous chemicals that adversely affect function in both developing and mature nervous tissue, are poisonous or destructive to nerve tissue, causing neurotoxicity. They are basically communication breakers; our bodies speak one language and neurotoxins speak another. Mercury, for example, has been found to penetrate and damage the blood-brain barrier, a highly selective semipermeable membrane barrier that separates circulating blood from the brain and the extracellular fluid in the central nervous system. It's like the door that separates the pilot from the passengers on an airplane. We want that door to remain closed during flight. If the pilots, acting as the brain of the flight, are distracted while trying to operate, then the function and safety of the plane could be compromised. The blood–brain barrier is like that door. In modern times, we've added high amounts of toxic chemicals, such as mercury, into our environment, which can easily pass through the doors of the blood-brain barrier and cause problems in the nervous system. Mercury is a naturally occurring heavy metal present in the air, soil, and water, and has been known to man and (also used in medicine) for millennia. But humans adapted it and started adding it to synthetic products, including pharmaceuticals such as metronidazole used to treat Lyme disease, as adjuvants in vaccines, and in amalgam fillings (also known as silver fillings). Today, neurotoxicity is indicated as a major cause of neurodegenerative diseases such as Alzheimer's disease. So what's the frontline treatment for neurodegerative disease in BioMed? Simple: Reduce toxicity. We need to identify the toxic cause and get rid of it, and we will explain how in a moment.

Toxins and the Endocrine System

Lastly, as if cancer and Alzheimer's disease weren't enough, when it comes to toxin-induced damage, we've saved the hardest-hit bioregulating system for last: the endocrine system. Interestingly, most of the toxins produced by petrochemicals are classified as xenoestrogens because they have a similar chemical structure to human estrogen. These synthetic estrogens, also called endocrine disruptors, mimic naturally occurring hormones in the body such as estrogens (the female sex hormone), androgens (the male sex hormone), and thyroid hormones (everyone's metabolic hormones). Sometimes they cause overstimulation—estrogen is a very powerful growth factor. Sometimes xenoestrogens bind to cell receptors, which blocks the naturally occurring hormones from binding. It's as if xenobiotics park their car in someone else's reserved spot (the receptor site). Then, the natural hormone tries to park but can't, because the site is full. When the natural hormone cannot get into the parking spot (receptor site), it cannot confer its normal signal and the body fails to respond properly.

The scary thing is, there are *lots* of these xenoestrogens floating around. A wide and varied range of substances are thought to cause endocrine disruption. They produce adverse developmental, reproductive, neurological, and immune effects in both humans and wildlife. In 2013, the Environmental Working Group—presenters of the annual Dirty Dozen list of high-pesticide foods—compiled a list of the twelve worst hormone disruptors. The list includes plasticizers such as bisphenol A (BPA), bleaching agents called dioxins, the agricultural atrazine, and flame retardants that cover clothing. Endocrine disruptors are found in many everyday products, including plastic bottles, metal food cans, coffee filters, detergents, couches, food, toys, cosmetics, and pesticides.

In addition, a 2008 Austrian study found that genetically modified foods (GMOs) damaged lab animals' ability to reproduce. The effects grew stronger in the third and fourth generations, suggesting that the great-granddaughter of a woman who eats GMOs could suffer infertility as a result. Results of this unpublished study were presented by University of Vienna professor Jurgen Zentek at an expert conference organized by the Austrian Agency for Health and Food Safety. In 2016, the CDC estimated that 12 percent of US women aged 15–44 experienced some form of impaired fertility, and almost one in six couples had difficulty conceiving.[8] A 2017 analysis published in the journal *Human Reproduction Update* found that, worldwide, sperm concentration in men has declined 52 percent and total sperm count has declined 59 percent over the forty-year period ending in 2011.[9] Meanwhile, the infertility services market, including infertility clinics, sperm banks, and fertility drugs, currently tops US$3.5 billion, up fourfold from twenty-five years ago.[10]

Today, the pharmaceutical industry simply suppresses or artificially overrides everything the chemical industry does to us. In the modern world it's not a question of *if* you are toxic, it's *how* toxic you are. We need to clean out the garage so our cars can pull in and out. If we don't do this, by the time we progress to chronic and degenerative illness, the body often doesn't have the strength to defend itself and eliminate the stored toxins.

Bioregulatory Medicine Addresses the Emunctories First

A fundamental premise of bioregulatory medicine is that the body's regulatory systems will function in a healthy manner when the burden of toxicity is removed. We change the oil in our cars every few thousand miles for the same reason we need to remove the toxicity from our bodies. For thousands of years Ayurvedic medicine has recommended a complex herbal cleansing regime at every seasonal change to clear the channels of the body of toxins built up over the previous season. Traditional Chinese medicine has used therapies such as cupping and acupuncture to help facilitate the detox process. European traditional medicine promotes liver cleanses at least two times each year. Why? Because toxicity is the primary cause of dysregulation, or blocked energy flow, and the oldest medical models have known this for a long time.

Bioregulatory medicine differs from allopathic, functional, and even naturopathic medicine when it comes to reducing toxic load, in two ways: first, in the order of events and second, in the choice of therapeutics. Where some complementary medicine practitioners are quick to throw natural detoxification-provoking agents around, before we can start pulling impregnated toxins out of stored tissues and the extracellular matrix, bioregulatory medicine not only tests levels of various toxins, but also ensures whatever toxins are present will have clear channels out of the body. If this clearing isn't done, then the patient could feel incredibly ill. It's like releasing a dam when there are fallen logs blocking the flow; you want a flowing river but not a flood. Stimulating detox without fully functioning emunctories is the primary reason many people report feeling sick when they either begin to lose weight or start a detox program. Toxins are released too quickly or they have no way to escape, so the body gets a toxic blast that can be quite dangerous given the unstable nature of so many types of toxins.

When the pace of detoxification does not exceed the capacity of emunctories to excrete toxins from the body then the aggravation, the healing crisis, can—and should—be avoided. Both before and during all detoxification-depuration procedures, all emunctory channels should be assessed and opened. If you are constipated, toxins can't move out of the body. The liver, kidneys, lungs, digestive tract, gallbladder, skin, and emotions are all involved with elimination. Elimination is also related to circulation and lymphatic flow. Everything is connected. Let's take a closer look at these emunctories and a few BioMed approaches used to ensure their function.

Intestines

The bowel works to cleanse our bodies of the food we eat that develops into fecal matter. It also eliminates toxic buildup that might come in the form of hormones, pollution, chemicals, or other harmful agents that the liver fails to process. When fecal matter becomes impacted in the bowel, the bowel might not perform at an optimal level, causing constipation and other digestive problems. What goes in must come out, and normal digestive health means having one or two formed bowel movements per day. Compare this number with the allopathic view of the need for only one movement every two or three days! Constipation can give rise to overgrowth of bad bacteria in the intestines, causing disorders such as small intestinal bacterial overgrowth. The use of edible and supplemental probiotics, enemas, colon hydrotherapy, and castor oil packs are just a few of the tools bioregulatory medicine doctors use before stimulating the release of toxins.

Kidneys/Bladder

Your kidneys play a very important role in the normal and everyday detoxification of your body. They have the job of processing nearly 180 liters (48 gallons) of blood every day. They filter, cleanse, reabsorb nutrients and water vital to the body, and excrete substances the body cannot use in the 1–2 liters (1–2 quarts) of daily urine produced. An overload of toxins can cause irritation and then the whole of the urinary tract becomes more prone to infection. When normal kidney function is altered, it can result in water retention, kidney stones, and mineral deficiencies. A diet high in sugar causes some people to retain salt and water, and it interferes with calcium metabolism contributing to weight increase and kidney stones. Adequate water intake, use of specific herbal combinations, and addressing protein levels (which we will discuss in chapter 5) are all supportive of kidney health.

Lungs

Breathing plays a critical role in elimination because—aside from the skin—the lungs are the first detox organ to be in contact with airborne toxins, chemicals, viruses, bacteria, and allergens. Avoiding all types of fumes and smoke is especially important for lung health, and this includes synthetic air fresheners and scented candles. For an effective cleansing of our lungs, we must learn to breathe the correct way, which is to make use of our diaphragm, allowing air to penetrate deeper into our lungs and lengthening the breathing process. Proper breathing involves taking long deep breaths and allowing the air to flow into our diaphragm, where our belly will blow up slightly, then holding for thirty seconds before releasing the air out. Use of various oxygen therapies also support lung health and function.

Skin

Our skin reflects our diet and lifestyle choices; it's essentially the mirror of our internal health. When the intestinal tract is dysregulated, we see it in our skin. When a heavy amount of toxins enters the body, the strength of our skin becomes weaker and therefore even more likely to allow toxins in. As the body cleanses itself during detoxification, toxins are pushed out of the skin from the inside, showing as rashes and other skin disruptions. Our skin is exposed to a variety of toxins from the environment and also from the products we expose it to. Cleaning out the cabinet of all toxic makeup, creams, lotions, shampoos, soaps, and perfumes and replacing them with natural products will help support the detoxification process. Dry skin brushing also helps to clear away dead skin and activate the lymphatic system. The lymphatic system supports every other system in the body, including the immune, digestive, detoxification, and nervous systems. In fact, poor lymph health underlies a host of conditions, from cellulite to cancer. Because the lymphatic system does not have a pump, we must stimulate the flow through dry skin brushing, exercise, and assisted lymphatic drainage.

Central Nervous System

From a bioregulatory medicine perspective, it's imperative to clear mental and emotional toxicity in order to stimulate healing. Many physiologic organs have corresponding emotional functions. In TCM, for example, the liver is related to anger, the lungs to anxiety, and the kidneys to fear. The emotional "signatures" of different organs are universal and are tied to biological systems. Toxic emotions include resentment, anger, hatred, guilt, bitterness, shame, sorrow, regret, jealousy, helplessness, depression, apathy, loneliness, fear, rejection, and the inability to forgive. If we cannot properly express or detoxify our bodies from these toxic emotions then they will impede the body's health. Bioregulatory medicine can help clear these emotions with tools that include neurofeedback, counseling, post-Jungian psychotherapies, and neo-Reichian therapeutic approaches, to name a few. By helping people to express their unprocessed emotions and to let go of negative thought patterns and self-limiting beliefs, bioregulatory medicine optimizes individual cognitive functioning, emotional management, and belief systems. Emotions are a type of discharge, and they need to happen. Crying, for example, is very healthy.

There has to be a way for toxins—emotional and chemical—to leave the body in order for healing to occur. Opening the way is the first step bioregulatory medicine takes to reduce toxic load. Once the channels of elimination are open, then it's time to begin biotherapeutic drainage. This is where the choice of therapeutics becomes highly unique, specialized, and personalized. Most importantly, all therapeutics are nature-based and produced using biological, not synthetic, means. This approach activates hormetic responses, signaling an appropriate response to evoke detoxification and discharge. Healing cannot even begin to occur until detoxification happens.

Biotherapeutic Drainage and Antihomotoxic Treatments

All treatments in bioregulatory medicine are intended to mimic, facilitate, stimulate, or promote the body's natural self-healing mechanisms. Detoxification is one of those self-healing mechanisms, that, as we've learned, can be dysregulated from overexposure to xenobiotics, nutrient depletion, and so forth. To counteract this dysregulation, biotherapeutic drainage—another core principle in bioregulatory medicine—utilizes multitarget treatments that act in concordance with multiple systems, feedback loops, and biorhythms. This is no over-the-counter herbal detox, but is rather a clinically monitored, whole-body, highly personalized, and specialized systemic approach of lowering toxicity and restoring homeostasis. Once the emunctory channels are open and the logs from our stream are removed, biotherapeutic drainage then facilitates and stimulates the discharge of toxic accumulations from the extracellular matrix, tissues, and organs. Biotherapeutic drainage treatments essentially shake up the cells and tissues, mobilizing and freeing the toxic sediments that settled on the bottom. Then it rids both intracellular and extracellular garbage on a physical, emotional, and energetic level, so the body can regenerate and heal.

There are three primary goals of antihomotoxic treatments: drain and detox, balance and restore the immune system, and provide support to damaged cells, tissues, and organs. To achieve these goals, some of the most commonly prescribed medicines are complex homeopathic remedies, also called homeotherapeuticals. Homeopathic medicine, first hinted at by Hippocrates and then further developed by Paracelsus and then Samuel Hahnemann during the eighteenth century, is natural biological medicine at its best, and comes only from natural sources, including minerals, metals, botanicals, or animals. Homeopathics are substances that our bodies and our genomes have coevolved with for centuries—naturally occurring substances with biologically active properties that are prepared through a series of dilutions, creating both an energetic and a therapeutic medicine to promote, facilitate, and stimulate drainage and healing. It takes therapeutics that act on both an energetic and a physiologic plane to dredge deeply rooted toxins out of cells where they've been comfortably seated for, in some cases, decades.

While allopathic drug development companies have been hard at work both creating and marketing synthetic drugs, homeopathic companies throughout Europe have been taking homeopathic medicine to the next level, creating highly specific compound formulas of plant constituents as well as glandular, hormonal, and immune compounds designed to target specific organs to facilitate the drainage of toxins, improve immune health, and repair damaged organs. Complex homeopathic remedies from companies such as Boiron, Heel, Pekana, Seroyal, Spagyros, Spenglersan, Wala, Weleda, and so forth harness the organ-binding affinity of certain plant compounds in order to drive pure potentized metal remedies into the cell, where they exert their pharmacodynamic functions that remove and drain both endogenous and exogenous toxins from target cells, tissues, and organs.

Homeopathic drainage remedies do many things. Not only do they have an active biological effect, but also they increase circulation, metabolism, and function in specific organ systems. For example, *Chelidonium* (celadine) and *Taraxacum* (dandelion) are liver-specific herbs, *Asparagus* and *Juniperus* (juniper) help the kidneys, *Valariana* (valerian) is for the nervous system, and *Verbascum* (mullein) supports the lungs. These biologics can be taken orally, injected subcutaneously, or administered intravenously. Complex homeopathic drainage formulas also stimulate and support normal metabolic processes that aid in detoxification and drainage, such as the Krebs cycle. (The Krebs cycle occurs in the mitochondria and is what generates cellular energy. This cycle gets bogged down when cells become overloaded with toxins, which explains why fatigue is the primary symptom in toxicity related to chronic and degenerative diseases.)

In addition to supporting the detoxification and drainage process using homeopathics, bioregulatory medicine also employs various other treatments, such as fasting, saunas, lymphatic drainage, minerals, tissue salts, spagyrics, immunometabolic remedies, and hydrotherapy (hot/cold), all of which help liberate toxins from deep tissues. Hyperbaric oxygen is also a powerful tool as it cleans the matrix while reducing tissue acidity and inflammation. Intravenous chelation therapy (*chelation* means "to grab" or "to bind") can also be helpful, and is the preferred medical treatment for reducing the toxic effects of heavy metals. Chelating agents are capable of binding to toxic metal ions, forming complex structures that are then excreted from the body faster than the toxins themselves. Use of natural compounds including 2,3-Dimercapto-1-propane-sulfonic acid (DMPS), alpha lipoic acid, and phospholipids can be powerful natural chelating agents. However, the practice and pace of chelation can be contraindicated if the emunctories are not fully functioning or if there is gut permeability, as released heavy metals can cross the blood-brain barrier and cause neurological symptoms. It's important to work with a trained bioregulatory medicine provider.

Allopathic medicine not only ignores toxicity, but also suppresses any type of drainage: Diarrhea is stopped, runny noses are dried up, immune systems are shut down. Yet stopping these types of drainage only causes side effects and fuels other pathologies. Bioregulatory medicine recognizes that the body naturally wants to and needs to eliminate toxins—for example, we vomit when we get food poisoning. Thus, BioMed draws on the world's most innovative technologies and biotherapeutics to help hasten the process, lighten the load, clean out the garage, and drain the disease barrel. Disease is not bad luck; in fact bioregulatory medicine practitioners can identify the evolution of it. And regardless of what disease a toxin caused, in bioregulatory medicine, the actual disease is not treated, per se, but rather the abnormal physiology is addressed, which is most often caused by toxin overload. Toxins, along with poor nutrition, dental infections, and imbalances in our nervous system, are what cause dysregulation and, ultimately, disease. We can reverse disease with bioregulatory medicine.

Next let's closely examine one of the most powerful bioregulating systems in the body: the digestive system. The food that goes into our mouths and ultimately into our digestive tracts can be either toxic or therapeutic. Therefore, nutrition is one of the most powerful tools bioregulatory medicine uses to restore homeostasis systemwide.

CHAPTER FIVE

Diet

Digestion, Nutrition, and Plant Medicine

When diet is wrong, medicine is of no use. When diet is correct, medicine is of no need.

—AYURVEDIC PROVERB

He that takes medicine and neglects diet, wastes the skill of the physician.

—CHINESE PROVERB

The doctor of the future will no longer treat the human frame with drugs, but rather will cure and prevent disease with nutrition.

—THOMAS EDISON

Many of us don't think much about food: how it was grown, how it ended up on our plate, what's in our morning granola bar. Sometimes, when things come easy, appreciation is lost. But for millions of years all humans had to actively search the Earth for food. Food was celebrated, ritualized, and prized. For most of human existence, the majority of waking hours were spent foraging edible plants and roots or chasing animals. There is fossil evidence of at least three species of hominids that were eating animal meat and marrow, in addition to a wide variety of fruit, leaves, flowers, bark, insects, roots, and tubers, starting around 2.6 million years ago.[1] The earliest evidence for hunting technology, spear points, dates back to about 500,000 years ago. By 164,000 years ago, modern humans were collecting and cooking shellfish, and by 90,000 years ago we had begun making special fishing tools. Then, within just the past 12,000 years—a mere comma in the novel of human existence—our species, *Homo sapiens*, made the transition from hunting and gathering natural, whole, wild plant and animal foods to producing, manufacturing, and domesticating our food sources. Over time, as our caloric and nutrient sources began to change, so, too, has our health. Our mitochondria started to see new fuel sources, such as grains, legumes, and cow dairy products. At this same the time, around 12,000 years ago, plagues became more rampant, and the stage for chronic illness was set.

During the past 150 years, we have witnessed the advent of man-made synthetic, genetically modified, biotoxic pesticide- and preservative-laden foods and beverages. Synthetically modified foods (*synbio* for short) are hitting the market in thousands of different forms—from genetically engineered salmon that grow twice as fast as wild fish to synthetic vanilla flavoring made using compounds found in coal. Like synthetic drugs, these foods are completely foreign to our DNA and also to our digestive and detoxification systems, bioregulating systems that evolved over millions of years to recognize, respond to, and require organic, carbon, and microbe- and nutrient-containing plants and animal food sources. Today, we not only are barraging our body systems with highly processed, biotoxic foods, we also no longer walk more than six miles on average per day in search of these life-sustaining calories. Today, calories are a twenty-four-hour convenience. Our evolutionary and genetic predisposition to move our bodies for food has been replaced by drive-through pickup windows. Both our food quality and food quantity have drastically changed, and these changes underlie the myriad of metabolic diseases, like diabetes, rampant in our time. Where once Hippocrates proclaimed food to be our medicine, in modern times food has become our biggest poison.

The poisonous potential of processed foods was first shown clinically during the 1930s and 1940s when Dr. Francis Pottenger published his famous cat studies. Pottenger observed that when cats were fed the same processed foods as people, they developed all the same diseases. A second group of cats was fed raw meat and did not develop all the disease that the processed-food-fed cats did. What's more, the processed food group all became infertile by the fourth generation of eating the processed foods, and it took four generations to reverse all these results. From this study, we can deduce that a major cause of infertility is a nutrient-devoid processed-food diet. And this situation can't be changed overnight with a multivitamin.

Food, as well as the befuddled concept of diet, has become a source of major confusion (and fodder for hundreds of best-selling books). For good reason: Food is spiced with contrast and confusion. We've heard that meat is bad, grains are good, fat is bad, milk is good. Two people eating together at a restaurant—depending on what they order—can experience two very different health effects from their dinners. One plate can have biotoxins like sugar, synthetic and artificial ingredients, rancid oils, and foods that many people have sensitivities to. Another plate might have foods, especially plant foods, that contain some of the richest sources of health-promoting macro-, micro-, and phytonutrients. The body processes and metabolizes an organic salad and pasta Alfredo very differently. What's more, food manufacturers have cleverly formulated our morning bowls of cereal to taste far better (read: sweeter) than a bowl of bitter greens. As a result, many of us have become addicted to processed food. And while we overeat calories, we are severely malnourished nutritionally. Most processed foods not only have a net zero nutritional value, they also contain antinutritional compounds that require nutrients such as calcium to neutralize them. For example, highly acidic foods such as candy and soda require buffering minerals in order to maintain homeostasis of the blood. Navigating the conflicting waters of what foods to eat (and sadly what foods we can afford) can be overwhelming. Making it harder still is the fact that many, often tasty, biotoxic foods that are banned in other countries remain legal in the United States—for example, artificial colorings such as Blue #2 and Yellow #5, the asthma-causing azodicarbonamide used to bleach flour, the carcinogenic preservatives butylated hydroxyanisole (BHA) and butylated hydroxytoluene (BHT). Genetically modified foods found mainly in corn- and soy-based products are also prohibited in most other developed countries but not in the United States. Meanwhile, these foreign and biotoxic ingredients are wreaking havoc on human homeostasis, bite by bite. Beyond digestion and detoxification, bioregulating systems including our immune and nervous systems are getting tossed off balance with every nibble of food that our genes don't recognize. After air and water, food is what has kept humans alive for millions of years. Today, it's one of the things making us sick.

As a result of toxic food, the prevalence of digestive disorders is ballooning. Digestive diseases encompass more than forty acute and chronic conditions of the gastrointestinal tract, ranging from common digestive disorders to serious, life-threatening diseases. Gastroesophageal reflux disease (GERD), celiac disease, Crohn's disease, ulcerative colitis, irritable bowel syndrome, diverticulitis, small intestinal bacterial overgrowth (SIBO), as well as digestive tract cancers, chronic constipation, and diarrhea have increased by over 30 percent since the early 1990s. An estimated 75 percent of Americans live with some type of digestive discomfort. The allopathic answer is, as always, drugs. For example, lansoprazole, a proton-pump inhibitor (PPI)—which has a warning label indication of two weeks or less of use—is recommended for long-term use by allopathic medical providers for many digestive complaints regardless of the warning label. Hiding in the shadows of multibillion-dollar revenues from PPI sales is the fact that, with their use, people's overall stroke risk is increased by 21 percent and risk of dementia is also increased. Yet PPIs have become one of the most commonly used classes of drugs in the United States, with fifteen million monthly prescriptions in 2015 for Nexium alone.[2] Other digestive disorders get similar allopathic treatment. Just Google "treatment for ulcerative colitis" and you'll see nonsteroidal anti-inflammatory drugs, antibiotics, immunosuppressive drugs, and surgical procedures such as colostomy and ileostomy. There's no mention of addressing the cause, which in most cases is the modern biotoxic, obesogenic, and highly inflammatory diet. Why? Follow the money.

In recent decades we've witnessed a significant crisscrossing and blurring of lines among the food, drug, chemical, and medical industries. Billions of dollars are spent each year by corporate food lobbyists, and government dietary guidelines have followed suit. Published in 1980, the food pyramid promoted low-fat diets with increased recommendations for carbohydrate consumption. We were fed a lie from the food industry, who said that fat is bad and grain-based carbohydrates are good. Despite the fact that humans have been eating animal and plant fats for millennia, in the early 1900s, chemicals and synthetic ingredients overtook our health care and food systems. Eggs became taboo, margarine a miracle. This change wasn't in the best interest of health; since 1980, when the government issued its first set of dietary guidelines, the number of Americans who are obese or have type 2 diabetes has more than doubled. Unfortunately, excessive absorption and accumulation of grain-derived carbohydrates leads to metabolic diseases such as obesity, hyperlipidemia, diabetes, and cancers. But allopathic medicine is right there to catch sick people when they fall, of course, treating them with pharmaceutical drugs. What we need, instead, is to clearly identify—and then change—harmful dietary habits. Meanwhile, the only "nutrition experts" allowed to work in most hospital settings are registered dietitians (RDs), allopaths of the food world, whose education derives directly from conventional commodity agricultural policies and special interests that subsidize cheap calories. Fast-food companies sponsor RD conferences, and corporate representatives give the presentation—special interest is rampant. It's time to start giving deserved recognition to nutrition therapists and other well-versed professionals who care about natural foods.

It's also time to start paying attention to our food and our food sources. Good medicine absolutely cannot ignore the primary importance of human nutrition—which also happens to be the oldest form of medicine. But if a poor diet keeps us sick, which in turn fuels our sick care system, there's little impetus in mainstream medicine to make a change. And so, the modern standard American diet, laden with common food allergens, sugars, processed carbohydrates, pesticides, and synthetic ingredients, continues to be the primary contributor to intestinal damage and permeability, weakened immunity, autoimmunity, and digestive disorders. While basic biochemistry shows us that poor diet disrupts homeostasis and promotes a chronic disease process, nutrition science is still not a required course in most medical schools today. Most allopathic doctors have a minimal understanding of nutrition, and so it is easy to see why nutrition is disregarded.

A primary focus for bioregulatory medical providers and nutrition therapists is reducing biotoxic foods from our diets while creating genetically customized biotherapeutic nutrition protocols. Healthy, nontoxic food choices promote drainage, reduce biotoxic load, and support the health of all of our bioregulating systems. In addition to placing a large focus on healthy foods and therapeutic doses of macro-, micro-, and phytonutrients, bioregulatory medicine providers and nutrition therapists also use many tools to determine the health of the digestive system and to evaluate nutritional deficiencies.

The tools include clinical assessments, laboratory analyses, bioresonance screenings, comprehensive stool analysis, HCL testing, pH testing, food allergy/sensitivity testing, intestinal permeability testing, bile acid assays, parasite testing, and bacteriology. All these tests, which are compulsory in bioregulatory medicine, are disregarded in allopathy. By contrast, to diagnose digestive disorders and diseases allopathy relies on highly invasive testing methods, including endoscopies (tube going down), colonoscopies (tube going up), and imaging such as X-rays. These tests are performed once symptoms present in the patient, and not before. Bioregulatory medicine tests for *prevention*, before disease has a chance to show up.

Dissecting Digestion

As Hippocrates said 2,500 years ago, "all disease begins in the gut." Wouldn't it be great if we could see everything that happened inside our bodies, and watch the magic of all the thousands of processes that occur within our digestive system? If we could peer at food as it's pulled down into our esophagus with the help of muscles that line our entire digestive tract—muscles that wave like a snake swallowing a mouse via contractions called peristalsis. If we could watch food as it is macerated by our teeth, then moves into our stomach where it swirls and churns like a washing machine, kneading that bite of food in with digestive juices into smaller and smaller bits, releasing nutrients. Imagine how what once was food is released by an arcade-game-like lever into the small intestine, our incredible intestinal lining activating immune complexes to identify the food particles, our intestinal microbes creating vitamins and facilitating nutrient absorption. What if we could observe the pancreas, squirting out secretions such as insulin and digestive enzymes that help the body utilize the macro- and micronutrients. And the liver, lord of metabolism and gatekeeper to all substances that enter the body, as it inspects all nutrients before the intestines absorb them. Indigestible fibrous residues (of which there are only a paltry few in the largely fiber-devoid Standard American diet) are fermented in the colon by a different set of bacteria that also help produce nutrients and energy. Now consider the synthetic foods we're eating today being processed by our guts, and the work our guts have to do in order to break down overprocessed materials that are downright toxic, and the overload of chemicals and the damage they do to the intestinal lining. Don't think food is all that important? Think again.

The Biological Importance of Human Nutrition

Biologically speaking, humans require food in order to derive the energy, structural materials, and regulating agents needed to support the growth, maintenance, and repair of all of the body's cells, tissues, and organs. Food provides so much more than calories. In order to maintain homeostasis, the human body requires the intake of over sixty different essential nutrients daily: thirty macro and trace minerals, thirteen fat- and water-soluble vitamins, nine essential amino acids, and three essential fatty acids. An *essential nutrient* is a nutrient required for normal body functioning that cannot be synthesized (made) by the body; we can't do without these essential nutrients and there are no other substances that can replace them. Essential nutrients, like tryptophan, magnesium, and alpha-linolenic acid, are the spark plugs of life. It's interesting to note that there are no essential carbohydrates in the list of essential nutrients, which is why low-carbohydrate ketogenic diets have been an important part of human evolution since the beginning of time.

Vitamins, minerals, and biologically active plant phytonutrients (*phyto* is from the Greek word for "plant") are primarily derived from plant foods, which are carbohydrates, and fruit- and vegetable-sourced carbohydrates are incredibly important in our diets. Grains and sugars are also carbohydrates but they contain antinutrient compounds and can even inhibit the absorption of other nutrients (including zinc) due to the presence of compounds including phytic acid. Some nutrients are considered nonessential, because in a perfect world our body is supposed to make them, as opposed to the essential nutrients that we need to consume in order to get them into our bodies. Vitamin D, for example, is synthesized by skin cells with the help of sunlight. Some conventional foods are fortified with vitamin D; however, fortified milk products have a nonbioavailable form of vitamin D, vitamin D_2, so it is ludicrous to think you—or your children—can absorb vitamin D from milk. Hence, over 80 percent of the population is deficient in this important vitamin. Required nutrients, including biotin, folate, and vitamin K, are made in your intestines by gastrointestinal bacteria; that is, unless you have a digestive disorder or microbial imbalance.

Nutritional deficiencies impair homeostatic equilibrium and eventually cause disease. There are 147 diseases known by medical science that can be induced, triggered, aggravated, or caused by calcium deficiency alone. Insomnia, muscle cramps, osteoporosis, hypertension, arthritis, Bell's palsy, kidney stones, colorectal cancer, premenstrual syndrome, gingivitis, and receding gums are just a few of them. In addition, zinc is needed as a catalyst for many enzymes; without zinc our metabolism would barely function. If your sense of smell or taste is lost or white spots appear on your nails, these can be an early sign of zinc deficiency. Adequate zinc, found in oysters, grass-fed beef, and spinach, is essential for adequate growth, immunocompetence, and neurobehavioral development, yet almost 25 percent of the world's population is deficient in zinc.[3] Has your doctor ever tested your zinc levels?

Magnesium, a mineral that activates over four hundred enzymes, is essential for blood vessel function, blood pressure regulation, and normal heart contractions. A deficiency in magnesium increases risk of conditions such as endothelial dysfunction, hypertension, and cardiac arrhythmias. Symptoms like constipation can inform us of a magnesium deficiency, just as bad breath can signal a vitamin B_3 deficiency. Dizziness and tinnitus are commonly caused by a manganese deficiency, whereas memory loss can come from a vitamin B_1 or omega-3 deficiency. Menstrual problems are attributed to vitamin B_6 deficiency, whereas slow wound healing is attributed to vitamin C deficiency. Varicose veins are caused by a copper deficiency; cardiomyopathy and thyroid disease from selenium deficiency; diabetes from chromium deficiency; and Alzheimer's disease from vitamin E deficiency (among other things). The list goes on, and on, and on. Nutrients are required for the bioregulation of every single system in the body. The human species evolved to require nutrients, and our bodies are also made up of all these nutrients. Our nutritional composition is a reflection of planet Earth in more ways than one.

The human body is one of the most complex structures in nature; many elements abundant on the Earth are also found inside the human body. Four elements make up more than 96 percent of our body weight: carbon, hydrogen, nitrogen, and oxygen. Similarly, all food-derived vitamins contain at least three of these elements (many contain all four). Minerals compose about 4 percent of the human body: Calcium, for example, is abundant in bone and teeth. This is why homeopathic medicine, which uses naturally occurring elements in microdoses, is so effective. We are born to run on nutrients, and there is no pharmaceutical drug that can ever replace their function.

Ensuring the body has the correct amounts of required nutrients—in the proper and most bioavailable forms (e.g., vitamin B_{12} in the form of methylcobalamin versus synthetic cyanocobalamin made with highly toxic cyanide)—is a fundamental tenet of bioregulatory nutrition. Creating homeostasis within a healthy body is like following a recipe. If you don't have the baking powder, then the bread won't rise. If you don't have amino acids, DNA can't be formed, nor can certain immune complexes. Conversely, an excess of certain nutrients can also backfire on homeostasis. Overconsumption of refined carbohydrates can cause type 2 diabetes. All bioregulatory systems require balance.

Orthomolecular medicine, a branch of bioregulatory medicine, is the practice of preventing and treating disease by providing the body with optimal amounts of nutrients, enzymes, hormones, and other molecules that are natural to the body. The field, practiced today around the globe and founded by two-time Nobel laureate American Linus Pauling, aims to restore the optimal environment of the body by correcting molecular imbalances on the basis of individual biochemistry. What's more, dietary supplements, including vitamins, minerals, essential fatty acids, amino acids, flavonoids, herbs, and phytonutrients, are the most valuable and safe substances for the prevention and treatment of chronic and degenerative illness.[4] Orthomolecular substances create the optimal molecular environment for our cells, improving metabolism and thus the ability of our cells to react.

Absorption and Nutritional Deficiencies

Once proper nutrition is in place, bioregulatory nutrition makes sure these nutrients actually get *absorbed*, and that the common deterrents to absorption are removed. In modern times especially, even though we eat nutrient-containing food we aren't guaranteed access to those nutrients when they are assimilated into our body system. Health is determined by what nutrients we can absorb. Many factors can contribute to malabsorption and nutritional deficiencies. For example, Americans typically eat 12 grams of fiber daily, less than half of what is recommended (20–30 grams per day) and half of what people ate 150 years ago. Inflammatory diets rich in sugar and processed foods, as well as certain medications and contracted infections, can contribute to nutrient deficiencies. Because of this, bioregulatory medicine prescribes optimal dosages for nutrients on a bioindividual basis, which in most cases are far higher than the recommended daily allowance. (The RDA, remember, are levels that are purported to prevent disease, not encourage optimal health.) There is a big difference between eating food sources of nutrients and taking supplements orally and even intravenously. For example, high-dosage, intravenous (IV) vitamin C (starting at 7.5 grams per IV) is used in BioMed clinics for cancer and other chronic cardiac and immune disorders. IV nutrition is a powerful and therapeutic tool because so many chronic and degenerative illness patients have compromised digestive function. In fact, one of the most common causes of nutrient deficiency is damaged intestinal walls. IV nutrition is able to get nutrients directly into the blood, bypassing the intestine, and in chronic illness cases, it is often the only treatment that can get patients out of the rabbit hole of chronic illness. But what causes damage to intestinal walls? A primary reason is the intake of food allergens and irritants and synthetic inflammatory foods, as well as medications, antibiotics, and chemotherapy agents—foods and substances that entered the human food supply in the past 12,000 years that our bodies don't recognize and therefore haven't evolved the proper detoxification and enzymatic response to. These foods include processed grains, sugar, genetically modified legumes, and denatured pasteurized dairy products. In the digestive tract these "foreign foods" are like a black belt karate master pummeling the endothelial lining that hasn't taken a day of martial arts training. Let's explore this a little further.

Intestinal Health and Foreign Food Sensitivities

Our digestive system—the intestine, liver, gallbladder, pancreas, and gut microbiota—is intricately linked to our neurological, endocrine, and, especially, immune systems. Digestion is crucial for breaking down food into nutrients, which the body uses for energy, growth, and cell repair. Food and drink must be converted into smaller molecules of nutrients before the blood can absorb them and carry them around to hungry cells throughout the body. This conversion primarily happens in the intestines. The intestine, including both the large and small intestines, is not only the biggest organ in the human body but also the most rapidly regenerating; intestinal regeneration can happen in as little as seven days. Recall that the most rapidly regenerating tissues and organs in our bodies (such as the intestinal walls, lymph cells, and intestinal bacteria) are the ones that hold the keys to homeostasis and vitality. The small intestine is one of these, and it has diverse biological roles, including nutrient absorption, barrier function, neurotransmitter production, and serving as an immunologic reservoir. In newborns, 98 percent of all immune cells are found in the intestinal walls; the amount drops to approximately 70 percent in adults. The mucosal lining of the intestine contains several antibodies known as immuno-globulins, including IgA, IgG, IgM, IgE, and secretory IgA. These immunoglobulins function as antibodies, activated, as you might recall, every time the body encounters any type of toxin. When this lining is damaged, immune function is compromised.

Once food is eaten, most of the absorption takes place in the small intestine. The inner surface of the small intestine is wrinkled into hundreds of folds and, when stretched out, is bigger than a tennis court. Each fold is contoured into thousands of ever-waving, sea-anemone-ish fingerlike projections called villi. Magnified more, each villus is composed of hundreds of cells covered with hairs called microvilli. Lymphatic and circulatory veins run through each villus, which contains enzymes that recognize different nutrients. Nutrient molecules either diffuse or are actively transported across the tight junctions of the intestinal villus cell membrane, entering the bloodstream or the lymphatic system. The complexity of our digestive tracts is astounding, and this complexity suggests the sig-nificance of obtaining nutrients.

If the microvilli are damaged or atrophied, the absorptive sur-face in the small intestines is reduced. It's as if a revolving door is spinning, and nutrients waiting at the entrance can't get in. Additionally, when these intestinal surfaces are damaged, the tight junctions that act as a protective barrier to keep unwanted particles out of the system also lose their integrity. This loss of integrity is called leaky gut, or increased intestinal permeability. In leaky gut, undigested food particles pass directly into the bloodstream, setting off immune reactions, and triggering numerous allergic reactions. Villous atrophy occurs when intestinal villi erode away, leaving a virtually flat surface on which nutrients are like soccer balls skipping across the ice rather than being slowed and absorbed by grass. Villous atrophy can result in serious nutritional deficiencies. Increased intestinal permeability, to varying degrees, is more common than most people realize. Bioregulatory medicine tests gut integrity so we know exactly—without having to go in and look—what is happening in there.

Celiac disease, for example, is an immune reaction characterized by damage of the small intestinal mucosa, and is caused by gliadin proteins found primarily in wheat, barley, and rye. Current estimates show that celiac disease impacts an estimated one in one hundred people, and rates have been dramatically increasing since the 1980s when wheat grains were first treated with the pesticide called glyposate. Today, wheat products such as bread, cereal, doughnuts, pasta, pizza, and cookies are the most commonly consumed foods in the United States. But villous atrophy can be caused by other conditions. There are documented cases of villous atrophy caused by cow's milk sensitivity, soy sensitivity, nut intolerance, opportunistic infections, intestinal lymphoma, ulcerative jejunitis, giardiasis, stongyloidiasis, coccidiosis, hookworm disease, leukemia, intestinal carcinoma, eosinophilic gastroenteritis, viral gastroenteritis, and drugs including methotrexate, olmesartan, Imuran, and Colcrys.[5] Vitamin and mineral intake can be negatively affected when phytates from dietary plant material (including cereal grains, corn, and rice) chelate and inhibit absorption.[6]

Many people are unaware that they have nutritional deficiencies, food sensitivities, or increased intestinal permeability but walk around with the classic symptoms. These symptoms include arthritis, diarrhea, constipation, depression, skin disruptions, congestion, difficulty breathing, headaches, and/or seasonal allergies. Sound familiar? Start looking at your diet; it holds the keys to health and disease. Bioregulatory medicine providers test micronutrient levels and address intestinal function and permeability in all chronic and degenerative disease cases. Testing for food allergies and sensitivities using genetic testing, electrodermal acupuncture, and serum lab tests is also commonplace in a BioMed protocol. All disease begins in the gut, so it's imperative to assess diet and digestive function together, as nutrient absorption can spell the difference between a cure and a chronic condition that does not end. In the words of Linus Pauling, PhD, "Provided one has the correct level of vitamin, mineral and nutritional input, the body can overcome disease." Proper nutrition is the prescription for self-healing.

Microbes, Genetics, and Bioregulation

While many vitamins and minerals that come from food are absorbed in the intestines, it is actually our gut microbiota that are responsible not only for the functioning of our immune systems, but also for the manufacture and utilization of many nutrients, provided they are intact. The human microbiome is emerging as having as much importance as—and possibly more importance than—our genes. Considered the forgotten organ, the gut microbiome, which hosts up to one thousand bacterial species that encode about five million genes, performs many of the functions required for human physiology and survival. It controls our immunity, metabolism, nutrition, and mitochondrial dynamics. In bioregulatory medicine, microbes stand at the forefront of treatment. And where allopathic medicine is quick to pull the antibiotic trigger against bacteria, bioregulatory medicine taps the wisdom of our microbiome to point toward the path of pathology. The true future of medicine will focus less on the disease itself and more on treating disorders of the human microbiome, which will in part be achieved by introducing targeted microbial species and therapeutic foods into our guts. The best drugs of the future will be full of friendly germs.

Bacteria

Humans coevolved with bacteria. And, like our body's mineral composition, our gut microbiota is a direct reflection of the microbes found in the Earth's soil. Just as we have unwittingly destroyed vital human gut microbes through antibiotic overuse, highly processed synthetic foods, and nondiverse diets, we have also recklessly devastated soil microbiota essential to plant health (read: the food we eat, the air we breathe) through overuse of certain chemical fertilizers, fungicides, herbicides, and pesticides. Soil microorganisms—particularly bacteria and fungi—cycle nutrients and water to plants, our crops, the sources of our food, and ultimately into our bodies. This is another reason why we are nutrient-depleted: Our food sources have lost much of their nutrient content in the past seventy-five years due to modern agriculture practices. Just because it looks like a tomato, doesn't mean it contains all the nutrients a tomato should have. "Reliable declines" in the amount of protein, calcium, phosphorus, iron, and vitamin C over the past half century have been recorded in forty-three different vegetables and fruits.[7] The average calcium levels in a dozen different vegetables have dropped by 27 percent, vitamin A levels by 21 percent, and vitamin C levels by 30 percent. If we work against nature in agriculture, we lose all of its bountiful health-generating effects.

Reintroducing the right bacteria, fungi, and nutrients into depleted and sterile soils with organic compost is analogous to eating prebiotic- and probiotic-rich foods (or taking targeted probiotic "drugs of the future"). Michael Pollan once stated that "the alarming increase in autoimmune diseases in the West might owe to a disruption in the ancient relationship between our bodies and their 'old friends'—the microbial symbionts with whom we coevolved."[8] We cannot deny the human connection to the planet, to the food we source from it, and the symbiosis in between. When we deny this connection, disease arises.

An estimated ten trillion bacteria call our gastrointestinal tract home; they vary in type and number, depending on pH, diet, and rate of peristalsis. BioMed practitioners want to know just what type of species of bacteria are in your gut, and in what amount, as many species need to be present in the right balance, or homeostasis is disrupted. Using state-of-the-art microbiome testing, bioregulatory medical providers can find out if you have the ideal population of specific strains, such as *Lactobacillus*, which helps with carbohydrate utilization, and *Bifidobacterium*, which neutralizes waste products and inhibits colonization of bad bacteria. These gut microbes are involved with protein, carbohydrate, and lipid (fat) utilization and metabolism by creating short chain fatty acids, the food of choice for epithelial cells to help facilitate fast regeneration. Vitamin K is produced by *E. coli*, vitamin B_{12} is produced by *Lactobacillus*, and folate acid is produced by lactic acid bacteria.

Microbes are involved with our brain-gut axis, which, when disrupted, is indicated in increased nervousness and many psychological and neurological diseases such as anxiety disorders, depression, and even multiple sclerosis. There is also an interrelation between the gut flora and the reactivity of a body to certain medications, including chemotherapy agents. Microbes are detoxifiers and deacidifiers, and, if all this were not enough, they also train and are intricately involved with the functioning of the immune system—including the processes of immunomodulation, immunostimulation, and immunosuppression. And just as biodiversity is important in the animal and plant kingdom, it is also important in our microbial populations. But, after millions of years, our modern lifestyle is putting our microbes on the endangered species list. As discussed earlier, our microbiome is formed during our first years of life, and early life exposures to foods, vaccines, antibiotics, steroid creams, inhalers, and more can influence our microbiome for the rest of our lives.

An overuse of antibiotics is of large concern in modern times. In 1945, an estimated 65 people were treated with antibiotics; by 2014, over 266 million outpatient antibiotic prescriptions were handed out. In 2016, a study in the *Journal of the American Medical Association* (*JAMA*) by the Centers for Disease Control and Prevention (CDC), in collaboration with Pew Charitable Trusts and other public health and medical experts, concluded that least 30 percent of antibiotics prescribed in the United States are unnecessary, and unfortunately, the rampant overuse of antibiotics (in food and medicine) is largely contributing to the public health crisis of antibiotic resistance. Today, drug-resistant infections are one of the greatest threats facing humanity. But antibiotics, in addition to antimicrobials, planned C-section births, reduction in breastfeeding, sterile environments, and toxic detergents, are resulting in a genocide of entire microbial populations. Add to these factors a low-fiber, high-sugar diet, hormone- and antibiotic-loaded meat and dairy products, excessive alcohol and coffee consumption, artificial sweeteners, and emulsifier-rich processed foods, and our bacteria populations are decimated and our intestinal walls are severely damaged. This is a recipe for gastrointestinal distress, nutritional deficiencies, and compromised immunity.

Homeostasis and the Acid-Alkaline Balance

The acid–alkaline balance (also known as the acid–base balance), the body's homeostatic balance between acidity and alkalinity, is also an important factor in bioregulatory medicine. The acid–alkaline balance of blood is precisely controlled by the body because even a minor deviation from the normal range can severely affect many organs and the ability to transport blood. Humans have several mechanisms that control our blood's acid-base balance, including the lungs, kidneys, and buffering systems, and we require a specific blood pH in order to maintain homeostasis of our body's many regulatory mechanistic systems. (The pH scale measures the level of acidity or alkalinity throughout various body tissues, blood, and the interstitial spaces, and the pH value is a number ranging between 1 and 14, with 7 as the middle point. Values below 7 indicate more acidity; values above indicate more alkalinity. While a pH of 7 is neutral, a slightly alkaline blood pH of 7.37–7.43 is considered optimal for human health.)

When blood pH is too acidic the body cannot respond or react, and healing is hindered. The proper balance between acids and bases in the extracellular fluid, the blood, and throughout the digestive tract is crucial for the normal physiology of the body, including cellular metabolism and microbial balance. Microorganisms grow best at whatever their optimal growth pH is—and some can tolerate more acidic environments while others can't. For example, when functioning properly, the parietal cells of the stomach secrete hydrochloric acid that brings the stomach pH to a range between 1.5 and 3.0. More than ten times more acidic than lemon juice, hydrochloric acid can burn straight through wood. Fortunately for us, the inner lining of the stomach is protected from its own acid by a thick layer of mucous and epithelial cells that produce an alkylating bicarbonate solution that neutralizes the acid. It's important that the stomach has a highly acidic environment in order to begin to break down proteins and release minerals, including calcium, magnesium, zinc, and manganese, while also inhibiting pathogenic bacteria or parasitic overgrowth. And this process is why acid-blocking medications do *not* cure digestive issues; in fact, it's estimated that approximately 90 percent of acid reflux cases are actually caused by low levels of stomach acid, not high levels.

Stomach acidity drops to a pH of around 6 at the start of the small intestine, then gradually increases to about a pH of 7.4 by its end. A vaginal pH of 3.5–4.5 indicates that there is a perfect amount of good bacteria (*Lactobacilli*), and no overgrowth of bad bacteria. Our kidneys do most of the work in controlling the body's pH by maintaining buffering mineral, or electrolyte, levels. When acid levels get too high, buffering minerals are called to action. These include calcium, magnesium, sodium, potassium, zinc, manganese, chromium, selenium, iron, and copper—all key to maintaining proper pH of the body. This is why calcium carbonate, the active ingredient in Tums, is used to rapidly decrease symptoms of an acidic stomach. And this is also why osteoporosis is so rampant in the United States today: When we consume highly acidic foods and beverages, such as sugar, processed foods, cow's milk, alcohol, excess animal protein, soda, coffee, and caffeinated drinks like Red Bull, the body uses its buffering minerals in order to neutralize them and maintain the correct blood pH.

When pH is imbalanced, an accumulation of cartilage-damaging acid deposits can occur in the joints and wrists. Uric acid, a by-product of protein metabolism, builds up in the form of crystals, like broken glass, and impregnates the feet, hands, knees, and back. This feels like gouty arthritis or joint pain. The answer to osteoporosis and arthritis is not drugs, however, but rather decreasing acidity in the diet and improving nutrition.

pH levels can be assessed via blood markers, via urine, and also via dark-field microscopy, also called a live blood analysis, which uses a high-resolution dark-field microscope to observe live blood cells and provide additional information about our biological terrain. It shows light images against a dark background—as opposed to bright-field microscopy, the conventional technique, which shows colors of a specimen appearing darker against a bright background. Like looking at stars at night, dark-field microscopy shows many components present in the blood that bright-field microscopy (like trying to views stars in the daytime) can't. Live bacteria, for example, are best viewed with a dark-field microscope. Live blood can indirectly show the presence of toxins or other blockages, white blood cell function, undigested fats, yeasts, heavy-metal toxicities, nutrient deficiencies, various bacteria and parasites, and the buffering load on the blood. While not commonly used, this is another tool that can help determine what is causing chronic pain.

Before we move on, let's focus on one important food: animal protein. The human species evolved eating animal meat, the only source of complete protein (meaning it contains all nine essential amino acids). Protein is important to human physiology; among many functions, amino acids are involved with helping repair a damaged intestinal lining, forming immune complexes, and facilitating DNA formation. These are just a few of the reasons why protein is considered a macronutrient—it is needed in large amounts, along with fats and carbohydrates—to maintain homeostasis in the body. But, just like all things good, we humans have taken meat, an evolutionarily advantageous substance (like sugar), and have been overconsuming it. An adult's daily protein intake should be between 40 and 60 grams as opposed to 140 grams, which is currently the average modern intake. For reference, one chicken egg contains 6 grams of protein, whereas an 18-ounce steak has 132 grams. So while consumption of protein is important, over-consumption can cause uric acid deposits in the interstitium and the tissues, causing clogs and hyperacidity. Too much protein can also reduce mitochondrial activity, causing fatigue, and can stimulate cancer-promoting growth pathways like mTOR. Most patients with degenerative diseases are actually hyperproteinized. Increased acidity and toxic accumulation create a less-reactive matrix that blocks informational flow between neurons and neurotransmitters. For some people, avoiding animal protein for a period of time to unclog the river is highly indicated. For everyone, avoiding highly toxic industrial meat that was treated with antibiotics and hormones and raised on a genetically modified grain diet is requisite to maintain health. Ask your bioregulatory nutritionist about your bioindividual protein requirements.

Overacidity, the Mesenchyme, and BioMed Treatments

As a whole, excluding acid-forming foods and drinks from one's diet, such as white bread, sugar, and supersized double burgers, is an important first step in supporting homeostasis. Simultaneously, the importance of regular intake of alkaline foods, such as green vegetables, is key for replacing those important buffering minerals. And by the way, sardines and collard greens have much higher amounts of bioavailable calcium than cow's milk (promotion of milk as calcium-rich is another food industry/dietary guidelines marketing scam). Addressing the effect hyperacidity has on the internal milieu is primary, so in some cases intravenous or targeted intracellular treatments are prescribed on a highly individual basis. Because the bioregulatory terrain consists of mesenchymal fluid and is the primary area of the body where communication takes place, an imbalanced pH can change the electromagnetic charge of the mesenchyme, which in turn disrupts communication. And because our bodies depend on the mesenchymal fluid to be intact in order to adapt, keeping protein levels in balance is critical.

In BioMed, one of the primary goals of treatment is restoring a balanced pH in the body. This is accomplished using orthomolecular medicine with particular focus on mineral status optimization and the use of isopathic and homeopathic remedies. All these treatments have highly effective results on regulatory processes like pH balance, the internal milieu, immune response capacity, and regulating the bacterial ecology within the body. Isopathy (*isos pathos*, or "equal suffering," refers to the therapeutic use of the exact substance that causes an illness as a therapeutic tool for that same illness) is the principle underlying conventional immunotherapy, and is a more specific subversion of homeopathic medicine. Sanum homeopathic isopathic and immunomodulator remedies have been used, with excellent success, by European health care practitioners for decades, and these side-effect-free treatments are now available in bioregulatory medical clinics in the United States, too.

Phytotherapy: The Use of Plants as Medicine

Now that we've established what foods to avoid in order to keep pH balanced and avoid intestinal damage, it's time to take a closer look at the active biochemicals found in plant foods and botanical medicines. The theme here is that substances that have always been part of our diets and are naturally occurring on the Earth not only are required for health but also provide the most powerful medicine. No matter how intelligent mankind has become, we simply cannot improve upon the wisdom and biology of Mother Nature. Many people might be unaware that phytotherapy, also called plant-based medicine or herbalism, dates back as far as the Neanderthal period. Today, in Germany, Austria, and Switzerland, phytotherapy is classified as a regular discipline of natural orthodox science-oriented medicine. At least 30 percent of today's pharmaceutical drugs are derived from plants. The broad, multifaceted reach of bioregulatory medicine also extends into the medicinal power of plants, drawing on the thousands of years of knowledge from Chinese, Ayurvedic, and European medicine traditions.

The power of what we eat goes far beyond providing required macro- and micronutrients; many plant foods contain chemicals that also convey medicinal actions. Plant medicine has been around for a long time—for as long as we have existed. The oldest written evidence of medicinal plants' usage in preparation of drugs was found on a Sumerian clay slab from Nagpur, which is approximately five thousand years old. It contained twelve recipes for drug preparations and mentioned over 250 plants including poppy, henbane, and mandrake.[9] There is textual and archaeological evidence that both frankincense and myrrh were used as medicinal substances in antiquity. Both frankincense and myrrh are tree saps, tapped from the *Boswellia sacra* and *Commiphora* trees, respectively. Frankincense (*Boswellia*) was historically burned as incense, while myrrh made its way into medicine and even perfume. Modern science has discovered that molecules in myrrh act on the brain's opioid receptors, explaining its pain-killing action, and the active ingredient in frankincense, boswellic acid, has anti-inflammatory and antiarthritic effects.

Herbal medicine, the central tenet of traditional Chinese medicine, Ayurveda, Native American medicine, and European traditional medicine—and of course bioregulatory medicine—is highly powerful on both a physical and a spiritual plane. The almost ten thousand different phytochemicals identified to date are chemical compounds that give plants their distinct color, odor, or flavor. Clinical data has found that phytochemicals can provide particular health or medical benefits, including:

- As antioxidants
- In immune regulation
- As anti-inflammatories
- In hormone modulation
- In tumor cytotoxicity
- As anti-angiogenics
- As chemopreventives

- In induction of apoptosis
- To inhibit metastasis
- To support DNA methylation and epigenetics[10]

There are three main phytochemical families: polyphenols, terpenes, and alkaloids. Curcumin, for example, is a polyphenol derived from turmeric root and belonging to the ginger family. It has a long history of use in Ayurvedic and Unani medicine to treat various diseases such as asthma, anorexia, coughing, hepatic diseases, diabetes, heart diseases, and Alzheimer's disease. Various scientific studies have shown that curcumin has anti-infectious, anti-inflammatory, antioxidant, hepatoprotective, thrombosuppressive, cardioprotective, antiarthritic, chemopreventive, and anticarcinogenic activities. It can suppress both initiation and progression stages of cancer, enhances the effectiveness of some chemotherapy agents, and has shown potential therapeutic benefit in experimental diabetes and hyperlipidemia studies. All this in just one bright orange root.

Various other polyphenols provide radiation protection from today's overexposure to electromagnetic fields and use of radiation therapy. Resveratrol, quercetin, and green tea polyphenols are among the top-studied and most potent radiation protectants in this class. Resveratrol, a natural polyphenolic compound produced by a variety of plants, such as grapes and some berries, is a radioprotector in healthy tissue and also has antitumor activity. Quercetin, found in onions, lovage, kale, and capers, protects lipids and proteins from otherwise lethal doses of gamma radiation, primarily through its antioxidant properties. Quercetin and other polyphenols not only provide chromosomal radioprotection, but also shield mitochondrial DNA from radiation-induced oxidant damage. Lastly, the polyphenol epigallocatechin gallate (derived from green tea) protects animals from whole-body radiation, blocking lipid oxidation and prolonging life span.

Terpenes, the phytochemicals found in plants and fungi, are the building blocks of complex plant hormones, pigments, and sterols. There are over thirty thousand different terpene structures that have anticancer, antimicrobial, antifungal, antiviral, anti-inflammatory, antiparasitic, and antihyperglycemic actions. Terpenes can be found in lavender, cinnamon, black pepper, tomatoes, rose hips, cannabinoids, and many healing mushrooms.

Mushrooms have a cross-cultural history of medicinal use spanning many millennia. In Asia, South America, Africa, and throughout Europe, mushrooms have been used medicinally and as food, as well as in rituals to awaken consciousness. Medicinal mushrooms have been used for centuries by Asian and European doctors and herbalists, and increasing evidence of their efficacy is making them acceptable to the Western mindset, as well. Studies suggest that specific mushrooms are strongly immunologic, help us maintain physiological homeostasis, restore physical balance, and improve our natural resistance to disease. More than 270 recognized species of mushrooms are known to have specific immunotherapeutic properties. In fact, medicinal mushrooms might hold the greatest immunological promise for the future of oncology and chronic infectious disease treatment.

Cordyceps, chaga, turkey tail, maitake, shiitake, agaricus, and reishi all contain terpenoids as well as other phytochemicals, including beta-glucans, polysaccharides, and ergosterols. Beta-glucans are known as biological response modifiers, and their ability to activate the immune system is well documented. Specifically, beta-glucans can stimulate macrophages, natural killer (NK) cells, T cells, and immune system cytokines. The medicinal mushroom *Agaricus blazei* Murill (AbM), originating from the Brazilian rain forest, has been long used in traditional South American medicine for the prevention and treatment of a wide range of diseases, including infection, allergy, and cancer. It has been demonstrated that AbM exhibits antimutagenic, antioxidant, and immunostimulatory activities. There are several reports from around the world of this mushroom being used successfully in late-stage cancers with otherwise hopeless prognoses. In fact, some European clinics base their entire treatment protocols on AbM mushroom extracts and other complementary botanicals. A 2004 study investigated the beneficial effects of daily consumption of an extract of AbM on immunological status and quality of life in cancer patients undergoing chemotherapy. NK cell activity was significantly higher after a six-week period compared with placebo. Additionally, chemotherapy-associated side effects such as appetite loss, alopecia, emotional instability, and general weakness were all improved. This white-trunked brown-lidded fungi is also showing efficacy as a remedy for arteriosclerosis, hepatitis, dermatitis, hyperlipidemia, and obesity. Integrating some extra shiitake, maitake, or chaga mushrooms into your daily diet or beverage routine will provide health benefits to you, so pick some up the next time you go grocery shopping!

Alkaloids, the third class of phytochemicals, are nitrogen-containing organic compounds with three thousand different types identified in more than four thousand plant species. Alkaloids and extracts from alkaloid-containing plants have been used for remedies, poisons, and psychoactive drugs for a long time. Well-known alkaloids, including morphine, quinine, nicotine, and ephedrine, and certain chemotherapy drugs, such as the taxanes paclitaxel and docetaxel, are derived from plant alkaloids. One alkaloid-containing plant that has demonstrated robust medicinal actions in particular is mistletoe, which attaches to and penetrates the branches of a tree or shrub, and then absorbs water and nutrients from its host plant. Though there are hundreds of species of mistletoe worldwide, only *Viscum album* is used to treat cancer. The scientific community has been studying mistletoe as an anticancer agent since the 1920s as its extracts have exhibited both cytotoxic and immunomodulatory properties. Currently, mistletoe extracts are used to treat a variety of conditions besides cancer, including HIV, hepatitis, and degenerative joint disease.

For thousands of years, mistletoe has been viewed as one of the most magical, mysterious, and sacred plants in nature. Mistletoe, or *Viscum*, was used by the Druids and the ancient Greeks, and appears in legend and folklore as a panacea. In Europe, injectable mistletoe extract was first used for cancer therapy in the 1920s by Rudolf Steiner and Ita Wegman, based on anthroposophical medicine principles. Oncologists have been prescribing mistletoe extracts for the past ninety years; by some estimates, 40 percent of French and up to 60 percent of German cancer patients receive this botanical extract.[11]

Every year, Germans alone spend more than $30 million on mistletoe preparations as cancer treatment. Results of a national survey conducted in Germany in 1995 by the Society for Biologic Cancer Defense found that mistletoe preparations were the most frequently prescribed botanical drug (80 percent) followed by trace elements, vitamins, enzymes, and xenogenic peptides like thymus preparations. In Germany, Switzerland, and Austria, mistletoe preparations are licensed medicines that are partly reimbursable through the official health care system. The US Food and Drug Administration, however, has not approved mistletoe as a treatment for cancer or any other medical condition. Fortunately for patients in the United States, some bioregulatory medical doctors are able to obtain injectable mistletoe extracts directly from Europe.

Unfortunately, mistletoe extracts are often given in late-stage cancer as a last resort after chemotherapy and radiation have failed. When started earlier in the disease process, mistletoe extracts such as *Iscador* convey impressive overall survival rates. Mistletoe extract is typically given by subcutaneous injection, usually one to three times per week, but can also be administered intravenously. In European clinics, a typical treatment course of mistletoe can last several months to several years. The doses are gradually increased and adjusted depending on the patient's general condition, sex, age, and type of cancer. For many US patients, however, the duration of *Iscador* treatment prescribed by US practitioners is frequently too short.

If you are suffering from chronic or degenerative illness, by now your doctor should have mentioned some or all of the following: frankincense, curcumin, medicinal mushrooms, quercetin, mistletoe, and maybe even cannabinoids. If they haven't, and you find yourself doing your own internet research, it's time you went to a BioMed clinic. While uses of these natural substances are powerful, they should not be self-prescribed. Remember, the dose makes the poison, and these natural substances are best used under medical supervision, because some can interfere with medications. Of course, there are many at-home bioregulatory practices you can and should start at once, beginning with getting back in tune with natural laws and adhering to a healthy diet that includes food sources of plant phytonutrients. But as with all things in bioregulatory medicine, there is no one diet, no one treatment, no one phytochemical that acts as a magic bullet. All dietary, homeopathic, and nutrient recommendations are custom-tailored to the individual, their genetics, and their health or disease process. When it comes to designing a therapeutic diet based on you, your terrain, and your disease process, consulting with a bioregulatory medical provider or nutritionist is critical. There are a wide variety—hundreds—of different diet possibilities, and thousands of books have been written on the subject. But diets *must* be adapted, to varying extents, to the individual. Anti-inflammatory, phytonutrient-rich, gluten-free, casein-free, paleo-type, ketogenic, or autoimmune diets are most often the base camps, and some amounts of protein restriction or variations on therapeutic fasting are also part of the biological medical therapeutic diet repertoire. Based on human evolutionary history, genealogy, and physiology, your diet should reflect what our Paleolithic ancestors (i.e., before agriculture) evolved eating over a million years and, as such, what has the highest potential of supporting healing and preventing disease.

When it comes to recommended therapeutic nutrition programs, bioregulatory medicine uses specific naturopathic, homeopathic, and/or herbal preparations with a hypoallergenic organic diet alongside intestinal cleansing. Apart from the use of probiotics, prebiotics, symbiotics, herbal tonics, and homeopathic preparations, all-around bioregulatory treatment for the digestive system also incorporates specific bioenergetics, psychosomatic, and structural therapeutic supports. Of note, once the digestive system is out of balance, it takes at least two to six months to reestablish a normal balance of the gastrointestinal tract and to reestablish insulin sensitivity. If there is severe insulin resistance or obesity, it could take much longer to stabilize. Yet most people will experience some improvements early on with a bioregulatory program. With time, our hope is you will notice less symptoms of your disorder and we will see improvements through lab values, blood pressures, energy, loss of weight (especially abdominal), and loss of carbohydrate cravings. Because food is often tied to emotional and neurological triggers, bioregulatory medical providers also address the psychosomatic elements of food relationships. Nothing is overlooked when it comes to reestablishing homeostasis of the body and the mind.

In the next chapter we explore the third pillar of bioregulatory medicine: mind-body medicine. We will explain the role of our nervous system in health and disease, personality, miasm, and constitution, and the energetic therapy tools used in bioregulatory medicine.

CHAPTER SIX

The Nervous System
Reuniting the Mind with Medicine

If you talk to your body, it will listen.
−BERNIE SIEGEL, MD

The moment you change your perception is the moment
you rewrite the chemistry of your body.
−BRUCE H. LIPTON, PHD

S tress comes in many forms: family worries, financial stress, marriage strains, pressure to keep up with the Joneses, global warming, politics, violence, toxin exposures, and, of course, anxiety related to health. In modern times the worries can seem downright endless. But stress is seen as standard, and never having enough time to relax is the norm. Who isn't "crazy busy"? These chronic stressors—stressors that don't seem to end—have increased in modern times. In 2017, over 50 percent of Americans surveyed reported experiencing significant mental stress.[1] Modern mental and emotional states for the majority of adults (and increasingly for children) include high stress, anxiety, depression, and neurological conditions including attention-deficit/hyperactivity disorder (ADHD), autism spectrum disorder, and Alzheimer's. Emotional, mental, and neurological imbalances, such as digestive disorders, are now so common they are almost accepted as typical. But in the Western allopathic medicine model stress has been grossly mistreated and ignored. Meanwhile, mental disorders are on the rise. Suicide rates are increasing. One in five adults is depressed. Anxiety disorders among teens are at an all-time high. There are currently more people dying from suicide than from traffic accidents, HIV infections, and substance abuse combined. Yet allopathic medicine continues to rely only on medications, such as thirty-year-old Prozac, which does not address the lifestyle, nutritional, biochemical, or even genetic imbalances that contribute to depression in the first place. So while physical degeneration has occurred in response to toxins and poor diet, our minds are becoming weakened as well. This is reflected in drug sales: The US population represents 4 percent of the world's population yet we consume more than 50 percent of the world's psychopharmaceuticals.[2] But do the drugs cure these imbalances? No: More commonly people become completely addicted to these mind-numbing medications, so much so that coming off of them can create a terror far worse than when they began. That's just not good medicine.

Our life stressors have certainly morphed from those of our human ancestors. Survival and reproduction—while indeed stressful—were the predominant everyday worries back then. The stress we feel—our thoughts—is something we can't see, and therefore it's difficult to measure or quantify. But even though thoughts and stress are somewhat invisible, they convey energy, and this energy has detrimental effects on all of our bioregulating systems, including the nervous, endocrine, and immune systems. When we become stressed, our levels of the stress hormone cortisol go up, and when those levels remain high, our risks of chronic inflammation, heart disease, and infectious disease increase. Emotions and behavior patterns create neuropathways in our brains and influence cell function. Descartes was wrong. His philosophical theory that the mind is separate from the body has been debunked over and over by modern science *and* it's been proven over and over that we sorely need to reunite the two. The mind and body *are* one. Bioregulatory medicine shines a beam of peaceful, restorative, and harmonic light onto our modern mental and emotional imbalances. For those stuck on the spinning wheel of chronic stress, past trauma, or neurological, endocrine, cardiovascular, immune, or digestive imbalance or disease, it's time to start paying attention to the role of the mind in medicine.

To heal from chronic and degenerative illness, medicine must dive beneath the surface of what we can see and measure. If illness were an iceberg, the visible floating tip would represent the clinically diagnosable symptoms. The vast submerged portion, often ten times larger than what we can see, would represent the mass of contributing factors, called the subclinical elements of a disease process. It's often what you *can't* see that is most important—and you can't see or quantify people's emotions. However, how we feel about, perceive, and respond to life stressors and events *does* matter. And in this chapter you will learn that it actually matters *a lot.* Stress, trauma, emotions, happiness—every experience we've ever had has created our unique biological biographies. These biographies affect our physiologies. A connection must be made between the mind and body for true healing, for radical remissions to occur. This connection is central to the bioregulatory approach.

Our cells and organs hold residues or memories within ourselves of everything that has ever happened to us. In fact, a massive body of research has shown that patients exposed to trauma-induced stress in their first eight years of life are more likely to develop mood disorders, psychotic disorders, posttraumatic stress disorder (PTSD), heart disease, dementia, high blood pressure, type 2 diabetes, obesity, and chronic pain than children who are not exposed to trauma.[3] Conversely, meditation has been proven to reduce symptoms of depression, anxiety, and pain. Research has also found that laughter can decrease stress hormones, reduce artery inflammation, and improve heart health.[4] Not only does laughter reduce stress hormones such as cortisol, but it also releases endorphins that can relieve physical pain while boosting the number of antibody-producing cells and enhancing the effectiveness of T cells. When was the last time you just breathed and thought of nothing for ten seconds? Or had a really good laugh? Or felt really happy, blissful even? If you can't think of a time, then it's time for a bioregulatory medicine checkup.

Mood or frame of mind, while somewhat transient, influences how we think and view the world. Mood is swayed like branches on a tree by more than just stressful life events; it's also affected by the amount of sleep we get, our nutrient levels, toxin exposures, hormones, even the weather. All these factors impact the triad of electrical (brain waves), architectural (brain structures), and neurochemical components that play in concert, singing our state of mind. The nervous system regulates mood chemicals such as dopamine, and it also controls bioregulatory functions such as heart rate. It's amazing anyone in medicine thinks we can separate the mind from the body. The same system regulates them both! This is basic biology. Just consider one of the best examples: the brain-gut connection. There is a reason why the gut is called our second brain. Our brain and gut are connected by a complex feedback loop of neurons, neurotransmitters, and hormones called the brain-gut axis. It's why people feel a pit in the stomach when they get scared.

Connections between Bioregulating Systems in Chronic Illness

Our brain is lined with a network of cellular elements that make up what's called the blood-brain barrier (BBB), creating a blockade between the bloodstream and the brain. The tight junctions that make up the BBB are strikingly similar to the tight junctions that line the digestive system, and are equally as important. Caused by the same factors that lead to leaky gut, the tight junctions in the BBB can also become permeable. A leaky gut leads to a leaky brain and increased permeability can allow any substance, including toxins and especially heavy metals, to cross over into the brain. Once this happens it is like the holes in a sieve getting bigger and bigger. In fact, digestive symptoms almost always present alongside neurological ones: headaches, cognitive decline, dementia, Alzheimer's, chronic fatigue, depression, and schizophrenia have proven roots in gastrointestinal inflammation.[5] A clinical review published in 2009 in the journal *Cardiovascular Psychiatry and Neurology* found that a breakdown in the BBB was observed in patients with major psychiatric illnesses, including depression and schizophrenia. Irritable bowel syndrome (IBS) has definitive links to anxiety.[6] We can't treat mental and neurological illness without treating the gut first, and vice versa. Using drugs to treat the mind is a medical approach stuck in the dark ages.

Specialized allopathic medicine is basically blind to the well-established psycho-neuro-endocrine-immune (PNEI) system, and the entire field of psychoneuroimmunoendocrinology. This fusion-focused field studies the interactions between psychiatry, neurology, endocrinology, and immunology. We know that the immune system is connected to the endocrine and neural systems via a number of pathways that integrate the functions of the hypothalamus, pituitary gland, adrenal glands, thyroid glands, gonads, and autonomic nervous system.[7] Recognition of these interrelationships gives bioregulatory medical providers the ability to apply medical knowledge to the treatment of different allergic, immune, autoimmune, rheumatic, digestive, endocrine, and cardiovascular pathologies. Do you have hormone imbalance, insomnia, or IBS? These conditions are all linked to a dysregulated PNEI.

The major area for improving PNEI-related chronic and degenerative diseases is psychological. In fact, emotional factors are the most common trigger of PNEI imbalance. Unexplained pain is almost always emotional. Low back pain, for example, often comes from a sense of supporting everyone else or a feeling of having no support. Several books have been published—including those from John Sarno, MD—that discuss how most back pain is emotionally based. In addition, cortisol and adrenaline are regularly increased in acute states of stress, a condition that, when prolonged, eventually taxes neurotransmitters such as serotonin, leading to insulin resistance, diabetes, weight gain, insomnia, and depression. Stressful states can also disturb the hypothalamus-pituitary axis, resulting in thyroid and weight problems. Sound familiar? Gut-brain, brain-hormone—all bioregulating systems are connected!

Improvement in stress management plays a crucial role in PNEI—and total body—regulation and homeostasis. For true health, we can't keep our emotions and past traumas hidden away in a box under the bed. Suppressed toxic emotions will eventually pop up as disease like a Jack-in-the-box. What is emotionally suppressed will be physically expressed. The body will *always* find a way to express emotional stressors. The body will talk through its symptoms even if you don't want to "go there."

The Nervous System:
Control Center of Total Body Health

The nervous system and its several subcategories are essentially a complex network of nerves. Nerves, or neurons, are cablelike bundles of fibers that transmit messages from one part of the body to another via electrical and chemical signals. The brain and spinal cord are considered the central nervous system (CNS), and all the nerves outside of them constitute the peripheral nervous system (PNS). Nerve cells in your fingers, for example, are part of the PNS. If your hand gets too close to a flame, the nerve cells in your fingers instantly transmit a message to your brain, the CNS, that in turn signals the hand to move away. The PNS is divided into two categories: the somatic nervous system (SNS) and the autonomic nervous system (ANS). The ANS regulates the functions of most all bioregulating systems, including the cardiovascular, respiratory, and digestive systems. In fact, the enteric nervous system (ENS), also known as the intrinsic nervous system, is one of the main divisions of the ANS and consists of a fishnetlike system of neurons that regulates the function of the gastrointestinal tract. The other divisions of the ANS are the parasympathetic nervous system, which controls homeostasis and is responsible for the body's rest-and-digest function, and the sympathetic nervous system, which controls the body's responses to a perceived threat and is responsible for the fight-or-flight response.

To summarize, the nervous system is the command, control, and communication center of the body that constantly responds and reacts to external emotional and environmental elements. If a loved one dies, emotional tear production begins in the limbic area of the brain where sadness is registered. What's interesting is that emotional tears contain different chemicals than reflex tears do. Reflex tears happen from peeling an onion, for example. Emotional tears contain compounds such as leucine-enkephalin, an endorphin found to reduce pain and improve mood. Yes, there is actual science showing the benefit of having a a good cry.

The brain produces neurochemicals including neuropeptides and neurotransmitters—such as dopamine, oxytocin, endorphins, serotonin, adrenaline, and GABA—to match emotions. In 1997, a brilliant molecular biologist considered the mother of psychoneuroimmunology, Candace Pert, published a groundbreaking book, *Molecules of Emotion*, that explained her discovery of the opiate receptor. This discovery changed the way scientists understand the mind-body connection, as these neuropeptides can alter both the mind and body. We all have receptors on each of our cells for neurochemicals, including immune cells. Neurochemicals connect to receptors like a lock and key, and cell receptors are the interface between emotions and the cell. When a neurochemical clicks into its matching cellular receptor, the resulting electrical charge changes the cell's electrical frequency and its chemistry. Like someone running into a house and yelling *Fire!* or *We won the lottery!* the mood inside the cell will change accordingly. The amount of receptors on a cell surface can increase or decrease depending on exposure. Cellular receptors increase to match prolonged emotions (grief, guilt, remorse, stress, heartache), and when these cells divide, they have more receptors of peptides for emotions. When cells are covered with many receptors for emotion peptides, those receptors can crowd out receptors for vitamins and minerals. This can contribute to early aging, nutrient deficiencies, hormone imbalance, and eventually disease. Emotions are stored in the body—and in our unconscious mind—via the release of neuropeptide ligands. These memories are held in receptors, which can alter energetic signaling, or qi, or life force—whatever you want to call it. Ever wonder why heart attacks are most common on Monday mornings?

If the sympathetic (otherwise known as the flight-or-flight) system is the gas pedal on a car, the parasympathetic system is the brakes. Prolonged stress is like having the gas pedal constantly pushed down, exhausting the engine and other mechanical features of the car. When we stop, or even slow down, we can take time to change the oil, change the tires, rest, digest, detox, rebuild immunity, regenerate, and heal. You can't fix a flat tire if you are driving ninety miles per hour down the German autobahn, just as the sympathetic nervous system is not designed to be used all the time. Humans are genetically designed to be in a parasympathetic state 40 percent of the time, but in modern times we far exceed this. Chemical stressors, as we discussed in chapter 4, cause a massive chemical stress response in the body. Over time, a chemically burdened, nutritionally depleted, and fast-paced lifestyle will manifest in chronic and degenerative disease. In addition, excessive stress results in mineral imbalances (sodium, potassium, magnesium) and manifests as fatigue, high blood pressure, and cardiovascular conditions such as palpitations, depression, anxiety, and dizziness. Turning to drugs results only in suppression of the symptoms, which is rather like lazy parenting. While there is a time and place to treat your child, giving a four-year-old a lollipop just so they can make it through a grocery shop only leads to a bigger meltdown later, or worse, total chaos when you refuse a lollipop the next time. At the end of the day, a functioning nervous system holds the key to both emotional and physiological regulation. And proper assessment is the first step. Bioregulatory medicine makes use of one of the most state-of-the-art testing methods when it comes to nervous system assessment: heart rate variability testing.

Heart Rate Variability Testing: The Gold Standard Multisystem Diagnostic

In under one minute, using no needles or other invasive testing methods, BioMed practitioners are able to evaluate the body's ability to adapt when it is under stress, and assess the functioning of the nervous system. Using a digital pulse analysis, heart rate variability (HRV) testing measures neurocardiac function, which reflects key heart-brain interactions and autonomic nervous system dynamics. You might ask, why are we testing the heart when we want to know about the brain? Neurocardiology research has shown that the heart is a sensory organ that receives and processes information. The nervous system within the heart (or "heart brain") enables it to learn, remember, and make functional decisions independent of the brain's cerebral cortex. Heart rate variability testing can show if someone is stuck in either sympathetic or parasympathetic tone and has lost their ability to adapt. A low HRV score, for example, correlates with higher likelihood of major depressive disorder, anxiety, inflammatory diseases such as Crohn's disease, adrenal insufficiency, and type 2 diabetes. This test can also show how well the heart is aging and how well it is functioning in response to stress. It is a nervous system assessment that has body-wide applications. Of note, there is no nervous system testing in allopathic medicine.

In allopathic medical offices, practitioners use cardiac-system-specific exercise or nuclear (meaning use of radioactive dye) "stress tests" to monitor changes in the heart's electrical activity and blood flow. These tests are limited to one system, and can cause side effects and obvious toxicity. If your heart function seems off, you get drugs from your cardiologist. If you are depressed, you get drugs from your psychologist. Yet broken-heart syndrome, Takotsubo cardiomyopathy (a sudden temporary weakening of the muscular portion of the heart), is a perfect example of the intimate relation between the brain and the heart as it mimics an acute coronary syndrome and can even result in sudden unexpected death.[8]

Some of you might be thinking, hold on, isn't all this health and disease stuff dictated by our genes anyway? And yes, in part, it is, which is why genetic testing is also an important component of bioregulatory medicine. However, the field of genetics has moved out of the DNA-dictates-destiny dark ages, into a field of scientific study called epigenetics. What we've learn in epigenetic research over the past thirty years has proven that there are vast arrays of molecular mechanisms that affect the activity of genes (think light switches), and these epigenetic "switches" can turn gene activity up or down. And guess what? Those switches are actually dictated by our environment.

Epigenetics and Biofields

Genes do not control us. They provide the blueprint for life, but our environment is the carpenter who actually builds the house. There is nature and there is nurture, and they are equally important. Yes, there are genetic origins in the variations of emotion processing, including mutations to the genes encoding catechol-O-methyltransferase (COMT), serotonin transporter (SLC6A4), and monoamine oxidase A (MAO-A), an enzyme involved in dopamine and serotonin metabolism. When these genes are mutated, people are more genetically predisposed to various mental illness. Yet we've learned that epigenetic processes, including methylation, acetylation, phosphorylation, ubiquitylation, and sumolyation—which are largely dependent on nutrients—control the volume of these genes. These epigenetic processes can also be impacted by heavy metals, pesticides, diesel exhaust, tobacco smoke, polycyclic aromatic hydrocarbons, hormones, radioactivity, viruses, bacteria, stress, trauma, and basic nutrients.[9] In fact, a wide variety of illnesses, behaviors, and other health indicators have some level of evidence linking them with epigenetic mechanisms, including cancers of almost all types, cognitive dysfunction, and respiratory, cardiovascular, reproductive, autoimmune, and neurobehavioral illnesses. To put it simply: It's not the genes that cause diseases, rather it's how our DNA responds to our unique environmental and emotional events. For example, a study in *Molecular Psychiatry* reported that children from impoverished families are more prone to mental illness due to alterations in their DNA structure. Poverty brings with it a number of different stressors, such as poor nutrition, increased prevalence of smoking, and the general struggle of trying to get by. All of these can affect a child's development, particularly in the brain, where the structure of areas involved in response to stress and decision making have been linked to low socioeconomic status.[10]

Environment is everything, and we are not separate from our surroundings. And while our nature- and nurture-based perceptions of stressors have much to do with our response to said stressors, it also has been shown that elements that enter our biofields have a big effect as well. We can't see biofields, they are a massless electromagnetic field of energy and information that surrounds, and is currently guiding, our biophysiological regulation. While the concept of biofields is "new" to Western science (the term *biofield* was only officially recognized in the early 1990s), ancient Chinese, Tibetan, Native American, African, and Ayurvedic medical models have recognized it for thousands of years. As the Hungarian biochemist and Nobel Prize winner Albert Szent-Gyorgyi said, "In every culture and in every medical tradition before ours, healing was accomplished by moving energy." But modern biofield therapies, including qigong, reiki, and therapeutic touch, have rapidly moved from fringe to forefront. These noninvasive therapies that work with energetics and biofields stimulate healing responses. And they work. So well, in fact, that the FDA has granted the use of pulsed electromagnetic fields for healing bone fractures and noninvasive brain stimulation devices to treat depression and migraines. Biofield-based concepts are also driving the multibillion-dollar global industry of neuromodulation, the use of externally applied electromagnetic signals for treatment of CNS-related disorders. Bioregulatory medicine has been on this bandwagon for a long time, making use of advanced medical device technologies that enhance or suppress activity of the nervous system by delivering nontoxic and painless electrical stimulation or natural agents to reversibly modify brain and nerve cell activity. Meet the chronic and degenerative disease cure additive of the future: biofield targeting.

Methodologies that are biofield-targeted include meditation, acupuncture, tai chi, homeopathy, flower essences and oils, anthroposophy, sound therapy, light therapy, healing touch, craniosacral therapy, qigong, and other new highly advanced technology including electromagnetic pulse and resonance repatterning devices. Energetic therapies all involve modification of the patient's biofield using external energies or vibrations, usually brought through the therapist's hands, with the use of machinery, or by the introduction of color, light, or sound. These therapies all have one thing in common: They acknowledge that a human being consists of a physical body capable of thoughts and emotions, but also has an energetic system that supports and nourishes physically, emotionally, and mentally. As we discussed earlier, the nervous system, the master control system, is *energy*. Therefore, energetic therapies are intended to improve the flow of energy and communication, helping to facilitate bioregulation. Energetic therapies are a very effective way to approach disease. Weak energy flow is like a poor Wi-Fi signal—the delivery of information is slow, incomplete, or distorted. Your hand can't pull away from the flame fast enough, or you can't remember things, or you feel depressed. The good news is you can change this without drugs, using biofeedback (a technique that can help patients gain more control over normally involuntary functions), perhaps the most well-known and widely used energetic therapy globally, as well as one of its subsidiaries, neurofeedback, which works specifically on the nervous system.

Neurofeedback: Brain-Training Treatment for Chronic and Degenerative Disease

Neurofeedback, also called neurotherapy or neurobiofeedback, is a type of biofeedback that uses real-time displays of brain activity to teach self-regulation of brain function. Biofeedback techniques can help patients gain control over normally involuntary functions like heart rate, and can prevent and treat conditions including migraine headaches, chronic pain, incontinence, and high blood pressure. These state-of-the-art, noninvasive, drugless methods teach the brain to function in a more balanced and healthful way. Neurofeedback is used often in bioregulatory medicine because it focuses on the central nervous system and the brain. Neurofeedback training has foundations in basic and applied neuroscience as well as data-based clinical practice. It takes into account behavioral, cognitive, and subjective aspects as well as brain activity.

Brain waves, including delta, theta, alpha, beta, and gamma, occur at various frequencies; some are fast, and some are quite slow. They are measured in cycles per second or hertz (Hz), named for German physicist Heinrich Rudolf Hertz, who was the first person to provide conclusive proof of the existence of electromagnetic waves. The brain, the body, and really everything has a measurable energetic vibrational frequency.

Gamma brain waves, for example, are very fast, with activity above 30 Hz, and are associated with focused attention, processing, and binding together information from different areas of the brain. Activity on the lower end of the brain-wave frequency band is associated with relaxed attentiveness, or alpha brain waves (8–12 Hz), which are slower and larger, and are generally associated with a state of relaxation. If you close your eyes and think of something peaceful like ocean waves, in less than thirty seconds alpha brain waves increase. Delta brain waves (0.5–3.5 Hz) are very slow and are what we experience in deep, restorative sleep. In general, different levels of awareness are associated with dominant brain-wave states. Thus, neurofeedback training is electroencephalogram (brain-wave) biofeedback. During a typical training, one or more electrodes are placed on the scalp and one or two are usually put on the earlobes. Then, high-tech electronic equipment provides real-time, instantaneous feedback (usually auditory and visual) about your brain-wave activity. The electrodes measure the electrical patterns coming from the brain, and your brain's electrical activity is relayed to the computer and recorded. Bioregulatory practitioners then map the brain and identify specific regions that are not working properly and, from that information, can directly retrain the electrical activity patterns in the brain. It doesn't hurt a bit, and the sessions are actually quite pleasant: You recline comfortably in a chair while sensors listen to your brain waves. A video, some music, or a game tells you when your brain is meeting the training target, and when it's not your brain guides you in the new reprogramming direction. Clinical research has shown that biofeedback therapy can be used to help prevent or alleviate conditions such as anxiety, chronic pain, insomnia, depression, high blood pressure, ADHD, PTSD, and more. Significant improvements seem to occur 75 to 80 percent of the time. Drugless, nontoxic, noninvasive, effective: That's bioregulatory medicine.

Neurofeedback is also being used increasingly to facilitate peak performance in "normal" individuals, executives, and athletes. Neurofeedback can help train the brain to become higher performing, and, like meditation, works with the brain to strengthen executive functions by increasing neuroplasticity. But neurofeedback is far from the only energy medicine technology we use in BioMed. Light, color, and sound therapies have also shown efficacy when it comes to chronic and degenerative disease.

Harnessing the Healing Potential of Light and Sound Energy

Light therapy—also known as phototherapy or heliotherapy— consists of exposure to daylight or to specific wavelengths of light using polychromatic polarized light, lasers, light-emitting diodes, fluorescent lamps, dichroic lamps, or very bright, full-spectrum light. In essence, it's the use of technology that mimics sunlight exposure, a natural law. Light is electromagnetic radiation, which is the fluctuation of electric and magnetic fields in nature. Light therapy is used in major hospitals to treat depression, seasonal affective disorder, and skin conditions. During light therapy, you might sit near or inside a device that emits bright light. Light is responsible for turning on the brain and the body, and enters the body through the eyes and skin. When even a single photon of light enters the eye, it lights up the entire brain. This light triggers the hypothalamus, which regulates all life-sustaining bodily functions, the autonomic nervous system, endocrine system, and pituitary gland. The hypothalamus is also responsible for our body's biological clock. It sends a message, by way of light, to the pineal gland, which is responsible for releasing melatonin, one of our most important hormones. The release of melatonin is directly related to light, darkness, colors, and the Earth's electromagnetic field. Light therapy is especially powerful for regulating endocrine disorders, including thyroid imbalances.

The ancient Ayurvedic physician Charaka, who lived in the sixth century BC, recommended sunlight to treat a variety of diseases. But the use of colors as a treatment also dates back to ancient Egyptians. In the hermetic traditions, ancient Egyptians and Greeks used colored minerals, stones, crystals, salves, and dyes as remedies and painted treatment sanctuaries in various shades of colors. Color was intrinsic to healing, which involved restoring balance. We know now why it works: because color is also energy, and light of varying wavelengths and frequency. Light is energy, and the phenomenon of color is a product of the interaction of energy and matter.

Colors are measured in terahertz, abbreviated THz, which is a unit of electromagnetic wave frequency equal to one trillion hertz (ten-to-the-twelfth power Hz). (Blue, for example, radiates at 606–668 THz.) Color is absorbed by the eyes, skin, skull, and our biofield, and the energy of color affects us on a neurological level. Clinically speaking, color therapy, also called chromotherapy, is a method of treatment that uses the visible spectrum of electromagnetic radiation to treat diseases, including cancer. Different colors affect different enzymatic reactions depending on the part of the body targeted.[11] Research has also confirmed that certain parts of the brain are not only light-sensitive but actually respond differently to different wavelengths. It is now believed that different wavelengths (i.e., colors) of radiation interact differently with the endocrine and nervous systems to stimulate or reduce neurochemical hormone production, including production of serotonin and melatonin. Colors generate electrical impulses and magnetic currents or fields of energy that are prime activators of the biochemical and hormonal processes in the human body, the stimulants or sedatives necessary to balance the entire system and its organs.

There are many different color-based therapies, including solarized water, light boxes/lamps with color filters, color silks, and hands-on healing using color.

Sound therapy is another healing method invoked by BioMed. In sound, or vibrational, healing, various sounds are used to detect and clear blockages in the biofield. The goal is to increase the flow of vital energies through and around the physical body. Vibrational energy healing, or harmonic healing, dates back to the ancient civilizations of the Lemurians, Aztecs, Egyptians, and Chinese. The term *vibroacoustic therapy* was coined in the 1980s by the Norwegian therapist and educator Olav Skille. Since then, research in Europe and throughout North America has shown that audio waves in the range of 30–120 Hz transmitted through a vibroacoustic device can have a positive effect on various systems of the body, producing a marked variable effect on heart rate, blood pressure, endocrine function, as well as metabolic changes. Vibroacoustic therapy has also been found in clinical research to improve the psychological symptoms of depression.[12] Sound therapy has been found to reduce the activity of the sympathetic nervous system, enhance circulation, promote cellular drainage, and even improve fibromyalgia symptoms. Just like color and light, sound is energy, and vibroacoustic therapy is based on the principle that life is vibration.

Indeed, all matter, including the human body, vibrates all the time, at various frequencies. Think of it this way: The human ear is capable of detecting sound waves ranging between approximately 20 Hz and

20,000 Hz, and the resonant frequency of humans is between 9 and 16 Hz. When various frequencies of sound are introduced to the human body, this vibrational medicine changes the frequency of the body, and acts as a catalyst to healing by transferring energy frequencies into the physical body to places where they can be most helpful. This process occurs primarily in the mesenchyme, which is the largely liquid and loosely organized mesodermal embryonic tissue that develops into connective and skeletal tissues, including blood and lymph.

Like Earth, our bodies are composed mainly of water—approximately 60 percent for an older person and 80 percent for a newborn baby. All of this water inside us is set into motion when the body is exposed to sound vibrations, like wind making waves on a pond. Vibroacoustic therapy is a safe, drug-free, noninvasive approach to reducing pain and anxiety and improving quality of life. There is also very strong evidence that types of sound therapies can shatter bacteria such as Lyme, destroy cancer cells, and treat hepatitis C. Furthermore many forms of industrial chronic and degenerative illness are thought to be the result from the effects of misharmonized vibration in the human body.[13]

Resonant Frequency, Quantum Physics, and Voltage Healing

Every object has a natural vibratory rate, or resonance. Every organ, every bone, every tissue, every system—all are in a constant state of vibration. In the 1920s, the highly controversial inventor Royal Rife created an "electromagnetic energy field" of a specific frequency, a concept that paved the way for what is now called resonant fre-quencies therapy. The concept of resonant frequency is based on the principle that a piece of glass will shatter when it is exposed to a noise that is the correct pitch. To actually break the glass, the vibration (coming from a person's voice or other source) has to match the vibration of the glass. If you "amp up" the volume of that particular vibration, the glass will eventually break. BioMed applies this clinically by matching the particular resonant frequency of living pathological cells, such as cancer, parasites, or bacteria, to the resonant frequency and then turning up the volume of highly specialized modern equipment. The cells shatter like glass, as the vibrations ensure that the molecules can no longer be held together. Over one hundred specific frequencies to various disease cells have been identified. One study used an oscillating pulsed electric field (OPEF) on pancreatic cancer cells and then later on leukemia cells. Pancreatic cancer cells were destroyed at between 100,000 and 300,000 Hz. For the leukemia cells, the procedure was able to destroy the cells before they had a chance to divide, killing an average of 25 to 40 percent of the leukemia cells and up to 60 percent in some cases.[14] Want to see this in action? Pull up the TED Talk "Shattering Cancer with Resonant Frequencies" from researcher Anthony Holland. It might shatter everything you've been taught to believe about medicine.

This concept has been proven by quantum physics. All matter, whether physical or chemical, is comprised of subatomic particles with positive and negative electrical charge. Therefore, we are electrical beings, and so is our universe and everything in it. Through these discoveries, it has been determined that every form of chemical or physical matter has a specific and measurable frequency, including everything that makes up who we are: organs, blood, the neuropeptides and neurotransmitters that we experience as emotions or thoughts, amino acids that construct our DNA, hormones that control and regulate our bodies, minerals, vitamins, fatty acids that feed our metabolism, and so on. Electrical energy is our life force. Therefore, the fundamental core of bioregulatory medicine is energetic therapies. It has to be. Healing is voltage. And this is why the energetic residues of natural substances found in homeopathic medicines are so powerful. (Of course, traditional Chinese medicine has known this for a very long time, which is why plants and herbs have been used for healing for centuries.)

The Energetics of Acupuncture

The basic premise of the healing modality acupuncture is that there is a vital energy (qi) that sustains the body and gives it life. This qi circulates throughout the body via a system of meridians, or what we call in BioMed highways of neurons. When some part of this energetic highway system gets blocked or overcharged because of physical, chemical, or emotional stress or trauma, then the body does not have what it needs to sustain proper health, and disease results. Messages can't get through, and so the hand remains on the flame, or the emergency rations can't get airdropped in. The acupuncture technique that has been most often studied scientifically involves penetrating specific points on the skin with thin, solid, metallic needles that are manipulated by the hands or via pressure, heat, or electrical stimulation. (Other acupoint stimulation techniques include manual massage, moxibustion or heat therapy, cupping, and the application of topical herbal medicines and linaments.) Acupuncture stimulates the central nervous system, which, in turn, releases chemicals into the muscles, spinal cord, and brain. A little pinprick says—*Hey, listen to me, over here! Send some rations in!* This then encourages a biochemical and neurological reactionary process that stimulates the body's natural healing abilities and promotes physical and emotional well-being. Case-controlled clinical studies have demonstrated acupuncture's effects on the nervous, endocrine, immune, cardiovascular, and digestive systems. By stimulating the body's various systems, acupuncture can help to resolve pain and depression and improve sleep, digestive function, and a general sense of well-being. A little can do quite a lot.

While the basis of bioregulatory medicine treatments lies in the centuries-old foundations of energy medicine, here is where the ultimate fine-tuning comes in. All these energy therapies utilized by bioregulatory physicians and therapists, especially homeopathics, anthroposophic remedies, essences of oils and flowers, and more, have to be customized or matched to the patient. Understanding a patient's personality type—what we call their constitution, miasm, or temperament—is the key to matching an energetic therapy to every individual's energetic resonance.

Miasm, Temperament, and Constitutional Types

Ever wonder why one person will laugh at a situation while another person cringes? In the movie *Parenthood*, Steve Martin is watching a school play where the kids turn chaotic, the stage falls down, and so forth. His mother-in-law is laughing her head off while he is sweating, gripping his seat, stressed to the max. Why? Because they have different temperaments. Let's go back a few thousand years for another example. The four temperaments or four humors theory can be traced back to ancient Greek medicine and philosophy, notably to the work of Hippocrates and Plato, who both had ideas about character and personality. In Greek medicine around 2,500 years ago it was believed that in order to maintain health, people needed an even balance of the four body fluids: blood, phlegm, yellow bile, and black bile. These four body fluids were linked to certain organs and illnesses and represented the temperaments, or humors (of personality) as they later became known.

The four temperaments became four fundamental personality types: sanguine, choleric, phlegmatic, and melancholic. Sanguine types tend to be enthusiastic, active, and social. They might thrive in sales and marketing positions. They tend to have good energy all day, but when tired they reach for sugar. Choleric types are independent, decisive, and goal-oriented, while melancholic types are typically analytical, detail-oriented, and deep thinkers and feelers. Phlegmatic types are relaxed, peaceful, and quiet. The phlegmatic temperament tends toward water retention and lymphatic stagnation, and they are slow starters, prone to chronic disease. A melancholic is a nervous type, who can be withdrawn and serious, and they are prone to acute illness; professions like accounting are attractive to them because they like to be by themselves. All these qualities are part of our emotional terrain. As we discussed in earlier chapters, from Hippocrates onward, this humoral theory was adopted by Greek, Roman, and Islamic physicians, and became the most commonly held view of the human body among European physicians until the advent of modern medical research in the nineteenth century. In fact, types of personalities have also been pervasive in various, more evolved, medical models. Practically all medical systems have their own constitutional typing. For example, traditional Chinese medicine denotes different types of people based on meridian or elemental expression (e.g., a lung, large intestine type, or a wood or metal type). Ayurvedic medicine has three personality types, also called doshas (vatta, pitta, and kapha). From the work of Carl Jung and Isabel Briggs Myers's typology, there are sixteen different personality types that refer to the psychological classification of different types of individuals. Good medicine should always match your type.

Hippocrates developed the four temperaments into a complete system of health and balance. Our unique human expression is the balance of these four qualities and defines our temperament. The four forces cooperate together to determine who you are, creating problems when out of balance and peace and harmony when in balance. A complete study of the four temperaments will reveal many unique characteristics, such as body shape, facial features, body fat location, personality traits, endocrine imbalances, libido, reaction to stress, career choices, food cravings, and others. Many homeopathic remedies are more appropriate for specific temperaments, such as *Calcarea carbonica* for phlegmatic types, sulfur for sanguinous types, *Lycopodium* for choleric types, and arsenicum album or silica for melancholic types. By balancing the four forces, one can improve health, character, romance, career, friendships, child-rearing, spiritual interests, and more. These energies ebb and flow in harmony or in competition, affecting every aspect of our lives. Everyone has one dominant humor, but all four humors are always present, whether blocked, diminished, excessive, or in equilibrium, and each humor refers to a type of fluid or flow in the body. The humors represent a powerful resonance between our selves and our environment.

Constitutional aspects are the characteristics of the internal self, our innate constitution given at birth. They can be defined as the functional habits of our body determined by our genetic, biochemical, and bioindividual physiological endowments, modified by environmental factors. In other words, the physical makeup of our body, including the mode of performance of its functions, the activity of its metabolic processes, the manner and degree of its reactions to stimuli, and its ability to resist the exposure to pathogenic organisms are determined by our constitution. In homeopathy, there is frequent reference to the "constitutional remedy" of a patient. Remedies are selected to match the patient's symptoms for a chronic condition, but particular emphasis is also given to their personality and temperament. Personality types are sometimes distinguished from personality traits, with the latter embodying a smaller grouping of behavioral tendencies.

A *miasm* is a reactional mode (i.e., a constitutionally ingrained pattern of reacting to stress and other forms of emotional and physical stimuli) that is bioenergetically transmitted from generation to generation. We were all born with energy patterns or miasms that were passed down from our parents. These energy patterns guide our physical, mental, and emotional interactions and reactions to the world. A miasm is the homeopathic concept of how the body reacts when exposed to something foreign such as bacteria, viruses, toxins, pesticides, or heavy metals and is transmitted from generation to generation bioenergetically rather than by the acknowledged genetic mechanism. The word *miasm* derives from the Greek word *miasma*, meaning "stain, pollution, or defilement." Dr. Samuel Hahnemann postulated the theory of miasms, noting that: "the disease would continue to progress [and] the remedies employed would do little or no good." After much deliberation upon this matter, he discovered that chronic diseases nearly always had a pattern that could be related to the presence of an imprinted miasm that both frustrated the action of well-selected remedies and impeded the process of cure. Medicine must match the disease, but to cure, it must also match the miasm.

A miasm is not an actual disease state, but rather a complex of constitutional characteristics and reactional tendencies that resemble the thematic pattern of the disease for which it is named. However, the influence of the miasm is how and why one person will develop a certain disease—for example, gout—while the same factors will cause another person to develop a totally different problem, such as an ulcer. Accordingly, each of the miasms has characteristic physical and mental emotional symptoms. This gave Hahnemann a reason to base remedy selection on the patient's underlying state versus the presenting symptoms. He made his prescriptions by taking into account the whole lives of his patients, observing what ailments they had throughout their lives and also observing their family histories. Everyone has an energy about him or her that will attract similar energies into his or her life, and this energy can manifest as a person, disease, or event. It's why people tend to attract the same kinds of friends, or partners, or become unhappy in every job. A person's reaction to anything foreign or new that occurs continuously in his or her life is most assuredly coming from his or her miasmic energy. This patterning determines each person's immune system reaction to anything foreign. All disease manifestations are expressions of miasms, regardless of their names. Thus, *miasm* is the term used to describe the predictable ways an organism reacts to challenges. The organism reacts due to its predisposition to different illnesses according to an evolution that is dependent on all the other factors that cause us to experience health challenges, such as diet, environment, stress, and poor sleep, which are all temperament issues.

This pattern is manageable with lifestyle changes and therapies, which is why bioregulatory medicine is so effective; it changes negative conscious and unconscious patterns. With use of therapies such as neurofeedback, flower and oil essences, single homeopathic remedies, oligotherapies, gemmotherapies, UNDA numbers, nosodes, energy work, and acupuncture (and all the therapies you will read more about in chapter 8), your biology *can* change. The assessment and management of a patient's lifestyle and history and the understanding and treatment of the patient's predisposition to illness (miasm), their temperament and constitution, are critical to be able to arrive at cure and, ultimately, to help a patient achieve wellness and healing.

The Medicinal Properties of Mindfulness

Prolonged psychological strain—from, for example, caring for a dying loved one, raising a child with emotional issues, a divorce that drags on, an overbearing friend, a job you dislike—is toxic by nature. These stressors are recognizable. Therefore, apart from somatic detoxification, bioregulatory medicine also supports a "psychological detoxification." By helping people express their unprocessed emotions and let go of negative thoughts patterns and self-limiting beliefs, BioMed optimizes individual cognitive functioning. Emotional and belief systems' management are approached using visualization, affirmations, progressive muscle relaxation, autogenic training, and meditation. Meditation and prayer offer big benefits to the balance within our nervous system. A balanced mind-body state can eventually decrease hypertension, certain heart conditions, fearful worries, inner tension, restless nervousness, distress, panic attacks, depression, addictive behaviors, and insomnia. We need time to be still, be quiet, and to envision positive outcomes. If you haven't yet, read Bruce Lipton's *The Biology of Belief*, Kelly Turner's *Radical Remission*, Bernie Siegal's *Clear Mind, Clear Medicine*, and Caroline Myss's *Anatomy of the Spirit* to better understand that what we believe is what we will perceive and how important our thoughts are. Attitude is everything. The placebo effect is not random, it is guided by thoughts, by believing a treatment will work, and embedded in what we know about neuroscience, biology, psychology, hypnosis, behavioral conditioning, and quantum physics.

We need to permit the body to relax, restore, replenish, repair, and regulate by allowing time to rest following daily routines. Feeling sad, stressed, or depressed? Studies have found that spending time outdoors can significantly reduce these feelings. Neurofeedback can also dramatically help. It is important to maintain a positive state of mind when faced with a chronic or degenerative illness, as optimism will impact your outcome. But time hurries us along, and diagnoses that are given a life expectancy or a time line manifest on a cellular level. Our biological clocks register these time lines. In the face of "bad news" it can be challenging, but we must try to reset our minds to live in the moment while remaining hopeful and positive about the future. We can't let time dominate our lives. If we give our bodies the feeling of endlessness, our cells will resonate with infinity and everlastingness. Time is just a way to organize everyday life and our professional contribution to everyday living; it used to be based on the sun, moon, and seasons, not the *second*. Physiologically, our modern construct of time can create stress, especially if we are running "short" of time. The body immediately reacts to the demand time creates. It speeds up our inner dialogue by sending out the wrong affirmations, like "I won't have all the time of the world." We need to be conscious of what makes us "tick," what fills our tank, and spend more time doing that. Arriving in the *now* will nurture the deeper awareness concerning our real needs and values. We need to give ourselves time to love, to recreate, to relax, to evaluate, to regenerate, to sleep, to do the things we love. Sometimes we need to *stop* in order to live. Living in the moment can be achieved with mind-body practices such as yoga, meditation, and tai chi and can produce effects including relaxation, reduced sympathetic arousal, self-regulated present-moment awareness, body awareness, positive reappraisal, and compassion for self and others, which can lead to improvements in physical and psychological health, and perceived quality of life. Yes, looking in the mirror every morning and saying: *I'm awesome*, actually does increase a feeling of well-being.

As we end this chapter, we'd like to assert that curing and healing are two very different things. Curing an illness doesn't mean that the emotional and psychological stressors and patterns that were a part of the illness process have been repatterned. This lack of repatterning is part of the reason why recurrences of disease can happen. The mind is the most powerful medicine, which is why BioMed uses many different diagnostic and treatment modalities to ensure the mind is balanced and optimally functioning. When we repattern our nervous system, our barrel is slowed from overflowing. We can't say it enough: *Our belief systems shape our biology*.

Next we'll jump into the last core tenet of bioregulatory medicine: dental health. Get ready to learn the huge, but largely unknown, difference between biological dentistry and allopathic dentistry. You'll never look at your biannual trip to the dentist the same way again.

CHAPTER SEVEN

The Mouth of Medicine
Mercury, Toothpaste Toxins, and the Oral Microbiome

The tongue can paint what the eye can't see.
—CHINESE PROVERB

Learning is like mercury, one of the most powerful and excellent things in the world in skillful hands; in unskillful, the most mischievous.
—ALEXANDER POPE

Your mouth does so much: smile, chew, talk, breathe, taste, digest. But, just as mental and emotional health has been plucked out of conventional medicine, so too have your teeth. Despite the fact that twenty-first-century science has firmly established that oral health is intrinsically and irrefutably connected with overall health, Western dentistry—and oral health in general— is kept completely separate from other aspects of allopathic medicine. Reuniting the mouth with the rest of the body is a fundamental tenet of bioregulatory medicine. This was recognized back in the 1920s, after Dr. William Gies—a Columbia University biochemistry professor credited with founding modern dental education—visited nearly every dental school in America and Canada and declared that dentistry must be considered a fundamental aspect of the health care system. As he put it, "Dentistry can no longer be accepted as mere tooth technology." He was right—oral health should not be separate from the rest of our biology. And in bioregulatory medicine, it's not.

By now, we hope to have driven home the point that medical specialization in one body part or system is just not the type of comprehensive approach required to meet the surge of chronic and degenerative illnesses facing modern humans. Oral health is no exception. Yet when it comes to specialization, oral health has been quarantined and farther removed from the body than any other branch of medicine. Divorced from medicine's education system, physician networks, medical records, and insurance and payment systems, a dentist is not just a specialized doctor but a different profession entirely. But the body didn't agree to this arrangement, and our teeth don't know they're supposed to keep their problems confined above the jaw. This separation between our mouth and the rest of our body can and does lead to negative consequences. An untreated tooth infection can spread to the brain, causing death, and only two hundred years ago, septicemia (blood poisoning) from tooth infection was a leading cause of death. A growing body of evidence has linked oral health, particularly periodontal (gum) disease, to several chronic and degenerative diseases, such as cardiovascular disease, which is the current number one killer in the United States.

Dental health is the missing link to overcoming so-called incurable diseases—especially the hard-to-diagnose type. Bioregulatory medicine not only embraces the role oral health plays in the concert of wellness, but welcomes it into the conversation of cure. The connection between dental infections and chronic, often vague, illness is so common that detailed dental examinations for those with complex illnesses should be requisite. Why? Because infected teeth act, as toxins do, as bioregulatory blockers, disrupting homeostasis. In fact, teeth are a common cause of remote illness in other organs. Dental infections can cause subclinical, local inflammation that interacts with various communication pathways, including bacterial, mesenchymal, and meridian pathways. Dental disturbances are often communicated throughout the body, and the rest of the body responds as best it is able.

Periodontal disease and hidden dental infections are common. As many as one in four people suffer from at least one, meaning approximately 25 percent of American adults have some form of chronic gum disease. Dental infection and chronic illness rates just about parallel each other. We absolutely have to close the gap between dental medicine and medicine for the rest of the body—and fast. Significant research shows the etiological and pathological links between dental disease and systemic, inflammatory conditions such as cardiovascular disease, type 2 diabetes mellitus, rheumatoid arthritis (RA), adverse pregnancy outcomes, cancer, and osteoporosis.[1] The link between RA and oral bacteria is currently attracting serious attention, bolstered by research revealing the complex interactions between the immune system and microbes in the mouth. In the BioMed health world, of course, we are not surprised. Consider this: What if the chronic pain epidemic plaguing modern humans has its primary origins in the mouth? Bioregulatory medicine—and modern research—knows that it does. And there's more, including adverse fertility outcomes. *Fusobacterium nucleatum*, an oral and periodontal pathogen, has been associated with preterm birth, stillbirth, neonatal sepsis, and preeclampsia.[2] When it comes to a healthy pregnancy, oral health is imperative.

In fact, substantiated relationships between dental infection and chronic disease have been confirmed a hundred times over. In the upper jaw, for example, the roots of the teeth are in close proximity to the maxillary sinuses. Chronic sinusitis (inflammation of the nasal sinuses), facial neuralgia, chronic eye disorders, and chronic or sudden-onset headaches can also stem from upper jaw inflammation. In 2011, Swedish researchers found that women are over eleven times more likely to suffer from breast cancer if they have missing teeth and gum disease. Every year more than a million people visit the emergency room for dental problems, and researchers have found that the number of people hospitalized for dental abscesses has increased by more than 40 percent between 2000 and 2008.[3] These folks commonly receive antibiotic and pain prescriptions and are then referred to their dentist. But many people don't have a dentist. For those that do, the mainstream view is that oral health is a surgical problem that needs to be drilled or removed rather than a systemic disease requiring prevention and holistic treatment.

In this chapter we will explain what happens inside your mouth, with particular focus on the microbes that inhabit it. Yes, the microbiome includes the mouth, not just the gut, and the mouth is one of the most microbially populated zones of the body. It needs to be, because the mouth is the body's largest orifice; every bite of food, medication, and sip of drink we swallow passes through our mouth. Therefore it *should* contain microbes—for immunity's sake. But in modern times these protective microbes are under siege, forced to morph from protective to pestilent in order to survive. We will also describe how downright toxic and synthetic our modern approach to oral care has become. How, in the name of oral health, we brush, swig, and are drilled with noxious chemicals including petroleum agents, bleaches, mercury, chlorine, fluoride, and nitrous oxide. The modern approach to oral care is akin to antibiotics for the mouth.

Bioregulatory medicine offers a holistic approach to oral care that utilizes novel diagnostic and treatment approaches, including safe amalgam filling removal. BioMed is a modern approach to oral health that recognizes the toxicity of the use of mercury—a proven neurotoxin in our mouths. The time has come to expose what the American Dental Association (ADA) has been trying to ignore: Mercury fillings are bad news for the body. Bioregulatory medicine believes that modern dentistry can and should tread as lightly as possible on a patient's biological terrain. Thus, a biocompatible approach to oral health is a hallmark of bioregulatory dentistry. But just how much do you know about your teeth? How about your tongue? Gums? Jaw? Many of us are only concerned that (a) our teeth don't hurt, and (b) the "social six" (the front six top teeth) look straight and white in photographs. But there is so much more going on behind those lips than meets the eye.

Open Up and Say Ahhhh: Oral Anatomy

Human teeth are the hardest substance in the human body, and they start forming around six weeks after conception. During the teething phase, little (painful) buds erupt into the developing jaw like tiny sprouts: ten buds on top and ten on the bottom—one for each baby tooth. These baby teeth are generally replaced by adult teeth between ages six and twelve. A normal adult mouth has thirty-two teeth total, which, except for wisdom teeth, typically erupt by age thirteen. Adults have eight incisor teeth, the middle-most four teeth on the upper and lower jaws, and four canines, the pointed teeth that are seated just outside the incisors and form the corner of the mouth. The eight premolars are between the canines, and eight molars hide in the rear of the mouth. Our four wisdom teeth are scheduled to emerge around age eighteen, but they are often surgically removed before then due to space issues or to prevent crowding of the other teeth.

Anthropologists believe that wisdom teeth were an evolutionary answer to our ancestors' early diet of hard-to-chew food like leaves, roots, nuts, and meats. Modern soft-food diets have not only changed our facial structure but also the space of our jaws; most of us don't need these extra molars to grind up pizza, pasta, and cake because these foods don't require much chewing. Our ancestors spent more than five hours a day *just* chewing their food to digest it.

Teeth themselves are made of a few different tissues. The hardest, white outer part of the tooth is called the enamel, which is mostly made of calcium phosphate, a rock-hard mineral. Beneath the enamel is dentin, a hard tissue that when damaged will trigger sensitivity or pain when exposed to extreme temperatures or pressure. What's called the pulp is the softer, living, inner structure of teeth. Blood vessels and nerves run through the pulp—the same blood that runs through the rest of our cardiovascular system, the same nerves that communicate with the rest of our nervous system. Our teeth are the only tissue in the body with just a single blood supply; every other bodily tissue has multiple arteries that supply needed blood, oxygen, and nutrients. A layer of connective tissue called cementum surrounds and binds the roots of the teeth—everything below the gum line that we can't see—firmly to the gums and jawbone. The periodontal ligament is a tissue that helps hold the teeth tightly against the jaw, and why our teeth don't wiggle unless we are about to lose them.

We're not much inclined to thinking of our teeth as living things, but the reality is that, like any other organ, they have a supply of nerves and blood vessels. When a tooth dies (most often from trauma or cavities) its pulp decomposes. As with an orange peel in a compost bin, decomposition by-products can be highly toxic and even carcinogenic. They include mercaptans, thioether, indol, and skatol, compounds that can cause an inflammatory reaction and trigger potential infection. Dental infections are tricky because there are not a lot of routes for these toxins to escape or drain. Inflammations are forced to swell through the apex and into the periodontal space, infiltrating ligaments and surrounding jawbone, which makes their treatment intensive and painful. When left untreated, infected and inflamed teeth are toxic time bombs. Yet until the infection is advanced, chances are you won't realize you have one.

There's a lot more happening inside your mouth than those pearly whites. Hundreds of small salivary glands secrete between 1 and 1.5 liters of saliva into your mouth during a twenty-four-hour period. Saliva is pretty important stuff. Approximately 98 percent water, the rest is comprised of electrolytes, proteins, enamel-protective nutrients, mucus, antibodies, microbes, hormones, mild, antibacterial compounds, and various enzymes including amylase, a digestive enzyme that converts starch into glucose (this is the enzyme that makes a saltine cracker mutate from salty to sweet in your mouth). The components in saliva are what control excessive plaque buildup and create the right microclimate for microbial balance to occur in the mouth. There are a lot of microbes in the mouth; up to 108 microorganisms have been detected per milliliter of saliva. *Streptococcus* is commonly found in saliva, and most of the time, when balanced, this bacterial strain lives benignly. But when out of balance, these same bacteria can cause strep throat, meningitis, and bacterial pneumonia. Balance, everywhere, is everything.

Most of us don't think too much about our saliva, until we don't have any. Trying to swallow a spoonful of nut butter with a dry mouth will elevate saliva to the "pretty important" list pretty fast. And spit is a spicy area in research, as there are important physiological hormonal activities that occur in saliva. For example, saliva contains peptide hormones, including epidermal growth factor (EGF), and amines such as melatonin, both involved in the regulation of inflammatory processes and the promotion of cell proliferation.[4] Less spit means less tumor-suppressive activity, and in addition to a reduction in important regulatory hormones, a dry mouth can have a negative effect on important oral microbes needed for immunity and digestion. The highly protective role of saliva might be surprising, but should not be underestimated. The most common causes of dry mouth include stress, cancer treatments such as chemotherapy, and many pharmaceutical medications, including antihistamines, antidepressants, blood pressure medications, antacids, and narcotic painkillers. When saliva output is lowered, it creates a systemwide alert—homeostasis becomes imbalanced. Two of the best ways to stimulate saliva production are to smell food cooking and, when eating, to chew food very well, at least twenty to thirty chews per bite of food. This complete mastication ensures the food is saturated in saliva. Eating with chopsticks or putting your fork down between each bite can help slow your gobble rate.

Speaking of surprises, the tongue, which allows us to talk, swallow, and taste food, is actually a key organ of the digestive system. The tongue is a mass of interwoven, striated muscles interspaced with glands, coated with mucous membranes and thousands of taste buds—sensory organs that allow us to experience the four primary tastes: sweet, salty, sour, and bitter. Beyond pleasure, taste enables us to evaluate foods for toxicity and nutrient content while preparing the body to metabolize foods after ingestion. Taste buds are rapid regenerators; they die and are replaced every two to three weeks.

The tongue has also long been known as the primary diagnostic communicator for the rest of the body. The ancient art of tongue diagnosis has been used for thousands of years in TCM. The tongue itself is considered a holographic map of the body's organs. During an oral examination (used widely in bioregulatory medicine), the very tip of the tongue reflects the heart, the lungs lie right behind the heart on the tongue tip, the spleen and stomach are represented dead center, and the health of the liver and gallbladder are depicted on the outside edges of both sides. Representation of the kidney, bladder, and intestines are on the farthest back area of the visible tongue, before it slips down the throat. Various dysregulations can be diagnosed based on the color and texture of the different parts of the tongue. A healthy tongue is pink, while a white-coated tongue might indicate *Candida* overgrowth. Vitamin B_{12} or iron deficiencies can turn the tongue strawberry red. A scalloped tongue, with ridges on the outside edge, indicates fluid retention. The tongue is the only organ that extends both into and outside of the body. It can see inside, and therefore it can provide a window into state of our internal health. Go ahead, have a look at yours.

While you are looking in the mirror at your tongue, take a flashlight and point it all the way to the back of your mouth. That is where the line of dentistry stops and other specialized medicine begins. There, at the end of the line, where the long tube of digestion plunges like a water slide downward, is where the pharyngeal tonsils (adenoids) live. The tonsils are vastly overlooked and underappreciated. As tissues of the oropharynx (the space behind the teeth, dark and forgotten) and parts of Waldeyer's ring, these two small glands house white blood cells and serve as the immune system's first line of defense against ingested or inhaled foreign pathogens, of which we have many in modern times. The tonsils provide a kind of guardian function—they can trap viruses and bacteria that enter the body through the mouth or the nose. They will become inflamed and infected when bacterial or viral populations become out of control. The tonsils harbor a unique set of microbes that, when out of balance, can drive bacterial tonsillitis and RA.[5] The typical allopathic treatment for chronically inflamed tonsils? A tonsillectomy, where both tonsils are surgically removed. This operation is usually performed by an otolaryngologist—an ear, nose, and throat (ENT) doctor—not a dentist whose scope of practice is limited to teeth and gums, nor an immunologist, nor a gastroenterologist. In medical specialty, the mouth has become a confusing place. But when it comes to oral health, the specialist who is really missing from the mix is a microbiologist. Microbiology is the most important element when it comes to not just dental but body-wide health.

Humans are host to billions of microbes, and the mouth is the mothership of many important bacterial strains. Removing tonsils, as opposed to identifying the underlying cause of imbalance (often bacterial), creates a systemic crisis for the immune system, as the protective bacterial front line is taken off the field.

The mouth houses the second most diverse microbial community in the body (the intestines house the first), harboring over seven hundred species of bacteria and somewhere between six billion and ten billion microorganisms that colonize the hard surfaces of teeth and the soft tissues of the oral mucosa. The oral microbiome is also sometimes referred to as the oral biofilm and, when in balance, is protective. The oral biofilm adheres bacteria to the teeth, which then excrete slimy sticky substances. Once these bacteria form disease-causing communities they become dangerous; their uncontrolled accumulation is the primary cause of cavities and gum disease. For this reason it is essential to disrupt "plaque" buildup at least every twenty-four hours, the approximate amount of time it takes for plaque to accrue enough mass and the bacteria to create enough acid to lower the local pH below 5.7, which results in tooth and gum damage. When in balance, many symbiotic functions exist between us and the bugs in our mouths, including antioxidant activity, maintaining a healthy digestive tract, resistance to colonization by pathogens, regulation of the cardiovascular system, and anti-inflammatory and immune benefits.[6] It is becoming increasingly clear that certain circumstances, for example when populations of digestive or oral microbes become unbalanced (more bad guys than good), can significantly contribute to the development of a variety of chronic and degenerative disorders and diseases. What causes the imbalance? Diet, in many cases.

Nutrition and Oral Health

Perhaps the best-known pioneer in holistic dentistry is Dr. Weston A. Price, dubbed the Isaac Newton of Nutrition. In his search for the causes of the dental decay he was seeing in his dental practice, Price traveled the world to study isolated human groups. He found that people who ate native, chiefly hunter-gatherer diets had straight, decay-free teeth. These traditional, largely pre-agricultural diets provide more calcium and other minerals, and fewer fermentable carbohydrates, which are the primary cause of tooth decay. Oral health stems directly from our diet. The mouth ideally maintains a neutral pH between 6.75 and 7.25. When we eat too many acidic foods, such as wine, sugar, or soda, the pH will drop, becoming more acidic—an environment that promotes pathogenic bacterial overgrowth.

Several common bacterial-driven problems plague our oral cavity, such as infected tonsils, mentioned above, and surgery is most often the only medical intervention. More than 530,000 tonsillectomies are performed annually in children younger than fifteen in the United States. Tooth decay (also called dental caries or cavities) occurs when plaque—an unbalanced accumulation of bacteria—grows on surfaces within the mouth, adhering to a tooth and producing acids that eat away at the tooth enamel by causing demineralization. It is as if your tooth were a Tums and you put it in a glass of water and vinegar. It bubbles away and eventually will dissolve completely. Cavities are, in fact, an infectious disease (the same disorder caused by organisms such as bacteria, viruses, fungi, or parasites in other sites of the body), and they are the most common in the world, affecting every population.

The typical treatment for these cavities is to fill them, and the content of many fillings is highly toxic (we'll discuss that in a moment). Gum disease, or periodontitis, is also a bacterial infection brought about by accumulations of bacterial-infested plaque in the mouth that eat away at the gum tissue and the ligaments that hold the teeth in place. Inflamed gums, or gingivitis, is a very common bacterial disease and the mildest form of periodontal disease. It is caused when a shift in the composition of the oral microbiome occurs and the mouth is no longer able to regulate itself. When the pulp chamber of a tooth becomes infected and fills up with bacteria, the nerves and pulp tissue become damaged. Severe infections commonly result in painful abscesses typically treated with oral surgery (an extraction) or a root canal, which can also confer toxicity (more on root canals later in this chapter). Halitosis, or bad breath, is often the result of unbalanced oral microbes that emit unpleasant-smelling gases. Have you detected the theme crawling across every one of these oral health conditions? It's bacteria. Bacterial balance holds the key to oral health and is why the oral microbiome is one of the hottest topics in medicine right now. So much of oral research is pointing us back to where we began: bacteria. Bacterial balance that is altered because of our diet!

Since the Agricultural and Industrial Revolutions, our oral microbes have witnessed significant changes. No longer chewing leaves and tubers, our oral microbes have had to adapt to pastries and soft drinks. Studies of calcified dental plaque samples from the time of our transition from hunter-gatherer to Neolithic societies and from the Industrial Revolution have shown both a compositional shift and a declining microbial diversity that occurred around both of these evolutionary milestones. For example, when we introduced grains to our diet in the early times of agriculture, certain oral bacteria had to genetically evolve their metabolisms to adapt to the higher-carbohydrate post-agricultural changes in our diet. *Streptococcus mutans*, for example, was able to successfully compete against other oral bacterial species by developing defenses against increased oxidative stress and resistance against the acidic by-products of increased carbohydrate metabolism. Sugar and fermentable carbohydrate consumption changes the composition of microbial communities, and they become dominated by acid-forming and acid-tolerant bacteria including *Streptococcus mutans*, which in turn produces more plaque and can become pathological. When homeostasis is disrupted, beneficial microbes transform themselves into pathogens in order to survive. Bacteria can change from one form into another, depending on the milieu, pH, protein content, trace elements, heavy metals, and so forth, in a process called pleomorphism. Thanks to the pioneering work of bioregulatory dentist Dr. Gerald Curatola and his book *The Mouth-Body Connection*, the importance of the oral microbiome can no longer be ignored.

There is no denying that humans live in intensive symbiosis with a world of bacteria that constantly changes according to the milieu, diet, and the acid-base condition of the person. As a consequence, bioregulatory medicine does not deem bacteria, viruses, and fungi as foreign to us, but rather as part of us. With this knowledge, we know that these potentially pathological microbes can be altered in their pathogenicity by correcting the inner milieu. It's not the germ; it's the terrain. Sadly, in the last 150 years, with surplus sugar in the Western diet combined with the advent of germ theory, our nuke-em-all approach to bacteria—especially in the mouth—has backfired, creating a pathogenic environment for oral bacteria.

Toxins in Your Toothpaste

Advances in oral care have traveled far from ancient Egypt, where dental creams and other breath-freshening agents were made by mixing powdered ashes of ox hooves with myrrh, burnt eggshells, pumice, and various grasses. During human evolution we've even been known to use solutions including turtle blood, human urine, and goat milk to deter halitosis (bad breath). Soap makers invented the toothpastes and mouthwashes we know today, which are basically flavored detergents used to wipe out bacteria and disinfect the mouth. The use of synthetic antibacterial agents in oral care happened as late as the 1800s. Listerine, for example, was originally invented as an antiseptic to clean operating rooms. Since the antimicrobial concept of oral care took hold, many studies have found that disinfecting the mouth kills the beneficial microbial communities required for oral health. Many oral hygiene products are basically antibiotics and pesticides for the mouth.

Most toothpastes have a poison warning on them—kids under age six shouldn't use them, and no one should swallow them. This is because there are many toxic ingredients in toothpaste and mouthwash, both substances we are all told to use at least twice a day. The fluoride in toothpaste and water sources is derived from a highly reactive element. We added it to the water supply in the 1950s to reduce an increasing rate of cavities (this was at a time when more people were consuming significantly more sugar, by the way). Disguised as a way to prevent cavities, the fluorosilic acid and sodium fluoride added to the water and our toothpastes are actually waste products from industrial fertilizers and other manufacturing processes! Anti-fluoride activists assert that water fluoridation allows the chemical industry to profit from creating toxic waste rather than paying for its proper disposal. The concept propelling its use is that fluoride will bind to tooth enamel, making it more resistant to bacterial acidification. However, we have learned that excessive fluoride can actually cause weakening of tooth enamel and bones, a condition called fluorosis. It's estimated that four out of ten adolescents have some level of fluorosis. Fluoride can also deposit in and cause calcification to the pineal gland, which is responsible for melatonin production and circadian rhythm regulation. What's more, fluoride has been recognized as one of twelve industrial chemicals known to cause developmental neurotoxicity in human beings.[7] It's time for doctors and dentists to get out of the chemical business.

Exposure to fluoride is suspected to impact nearly every part of the human body and the potential for harm has been clearly established in scientific research. A 2006 report by the National Research Council identified a number of health risks associated with fluoride exposure. Infants, children, and individuals with diabetes or renal or thyroid problems are known to be more severely impacted by intake of fluoride. A Chinese study found that drinking fluoridated water lowered IQs in children. Chlorine or hypochlorite, highly toxic substances, are used to kill certain bacteria and other microbes in tap water. Researchers have now linked chlorine in drinking water to higher incidences of bladder, rectal, and breast cancers. Reportedly chlorine, once in water, interacts with organic compounds to create trihalomethanes—which when ingested encourage the creation of free radicals that can destroy or damage vital cells in the body. Brushing your teeth with public water is far more toxic than you might realize. Bioregulatory medicine recommends drinking and brushing with filtered water, and preferably not bottled water, which adds a horrific amount of pollution into our ecosphere.

The cosmetic industry (the industry that covers oral care products) is largely able to police themselves under current regulations, and so armfuls of toxic or carcinogenic ingredients are commonly added to toothpaste in addition to fluoride, including: sodium lauryl sulfate, parabens, carrageenan, propylene glycol, diethanolamine, and microbeads. Artificial dyes and colors, derived from coal tar, have been linked to allergic reactions, headaches, and hyperactivity and related behavioral problems in children. Sodium lauryl sulfate, also known as sodium laureth sulfate, is a surfactant foaming agent that is also the active compound in some insecticides. The active ingredient found in antifreeze, propylene glycol, can promote organ issues, while diethanolamine, a foaming agent, has been linked with various cancers—and could be lurking in your toothpaste. And you don't even need to swallow these compounds for them to be absorbed through the lining of your cheeks. When it comes to oral—and body—care products, the golden rule is that if you can't eat it, don't use it.

Perhaps the biggest modern tooth-cleaning myth to debunk is the use of sugar alcohols in toothpaste. Xylitol and other sugar alcohols are the toothpaste equivalent of margarine. Nearly 80 percent of xylitol produced comes from genetically modified corn, is produced via hydrogenation, is deadly to dogs, is a metabolic disruptor, and can cause digestive complaints. Fortunately, several brands of toothpaste have been formulated to help support the health of oral microbes, including Revitin, Dr. Wolff's, Weleda, and Dr. Bronner's to name just a few.

The toxic element of oral care products is one thing; the fact that these products are not doing much to prevent tooth decay and infection is another. In 2014 the Centers for Disease Control and Prevention (CDC) estimated that 42 percent of children between the ages of two and eleven had cavities in baby teeth—numbers reaching epidemic proportions. It's not the toothpaste, in other words; there is an underlying cause. We are eating an unprecedented amount of sugar and fermentable carbohydrates—including processed grains, fruits, and fruit juices—which feed the type of bacteria that produce more plaque and then use oral care products that deplete the small amount of good microbes left. We take daily medications that deplete saliva. When all these factors add up—tooth decay, infections, and death of the tooth can ensue. When these conditions happen, they are largely treated with the dental version of an allopathic medical approach—root canals, mercury fillings, and even higher doses of fluoride. Now let's take a closer look at the conditions affecting our oral cavities and the mainstream dental treatment for them.

Hidden Toxicity in Oral Treatments

Conventional dentists don't talk enough about diet, rather choosing to mask the problem with highly toxic compounds and heavy metals, including mercury and endocrine disruptors like BPA. Dental amalgam fillings (*amalgam* meaning "a mixture or blend") are typically a combination of metals including mercury, silver, copper, nickel, tin, gold, and sometimes zinc. Also called silver fillings, most dental amalgams are approximately 50 percent elemental mercury. Mercury wasn't used in oral care until the fifteenth century; before that, silver and tin dental amalgams were first used by the Chinese, with evidence of use during in the Tang dynasty (AD 618–907). The problem is, scientific evidence has established beyond any doubt that amalgams release mercury in significant quantities, and that chronic exposure to mercury increases the risk of physiological harm. What's disconcerting is that all other mercurial medical devices and mercury-containing substances have been banned or removed from use, including mercurial wound disinfectants, mercurial diuretics, mercury in vaccines, mercury thermometers, and mercurial veterinary substances. Many other countries, including Germany, Canada, Norway, Sweden, and Denmark, have restricted or completely banned use of mercury in dental amalgam fillings. Mercury is forbidden in every other sphere of medical use and it has to be disposed of as toxic waste. So the question for the American Dental Association is this: How is mercury harmless in a patient's mouth? In an era when the public is advised to be concerned about mercury exposure through fish consumption, why aren't we told about the dangers of dental mercury amalgam fillings? Especially when more than 40 percent of all American dental offices are still using them. It is time to blow the whistle.

Various forms of heavy-metal toxicity, including mercury, are among the most widespread in the Western world—more so than nicotine and alcohol. When it comes to toxic effect, heavy metals are a primary cause of deep-reaching cellular disorders. Because a heavy-metal burden creates numerous symptoms, amalgam-related disease remains unrecognized by allopathic medicine. Symptoms of heavy-metal toxicity can present in a number of ways, including allergies, asthma, colitis, vaginal yeast infection, insomnia, chronic cough, headache, thyroid disorders, migraine, depressive mood, alopecia, eczemas, and more. Full-blown and typical "heavy-metal diseases" include multiple sclerosis, Parkinson's, chronic fatigue, chronic sinusitis, infertility, and ulcerative colitis. The symptoms of mercury poisoning and Alzheimer's disease are exactly the same. Something is very wrong here.

Mercury has an insidious affinity for mitochondria. Once it binds, mercury induces mitochondrial dysfunction, reducing ATP (energy) synthesis while increasing lipid, protein, and DNA peroxidation.[8] If that wasn't enough, this metal basically maims nutrients. Mercury is a selenium antagonist and blocks the intra-cellular function of zinc; both of these minerals are required for immune function and are fundamental cellular elements. Mercury also specifically competes with magnesium, interfering with all magnesium-dependent metabolic pathways including the produc-tion of energy from ATP.[9] This leads directly to a lack of chemical energy and also reduces the cell's ability to heal and regenerate. Signs of magnesium deficiency include confusion, depression, mus-cle cramps, constipation, abnormal heart rhythms, migraines, and seizures. Numerous illnesses have been associated with magnesium deficiency, including multiple sclerosis, hypertension, insulin resis-tance, diabetes mellitus, gluten-sensitive enteropathy, premenstrual mood changes, migraine, rheumatoid arthritis, arrhythmias, myo-cardial infarction, and sudden coronary death. Ninety percent of the world's anthropogenic mercury pollution comes from dental fillings, but we are also exposed to it in seafood (especially king mackerel, swordfish, shark, and tilefish), industrial sources, and even high-fructose corn syrup has been shown to contain trace amounts of mercury as a result of manufacturing processes.

Various factors can encourage the release of mercury from amalgam fillings, including acidic saliva caused by acidic foods like sugar, use of metal silverware, warm beverages, older fillings, EMFs, nicotine, bruxism, and mechanical overloading by chewing gum. Dental amalgams emit trace amounts of mercury, primarily in vapor form, which we then inhale. If two fillings are next to each other, and one is silver and one is gold, a galvanic (electrical) current will be formed between them, which can also encourage mercury to be pulled out at a more rapid rate. These oral galvanic currents created between various alloys in amalgam fillings—and that use saliva as a conductor—are highly disruptive to homeostasis. Like a battery, they produce currents that can interfere with electron flow. This communication disruption and increased release of mercury has such profound impact on homeostasis that bioregulatory dentists will measure dental currents using a galvanometer. As if these galvanic currents weren't enough, release of mercury from dental amalgam restorations is also increased after exposure to electromagnetic fields such as those generated by an MRI and cell phones.[10] You read correctly, using your cell phone close to a filling-filled face increases the release of neurotoxic mercury. It's time you knew.

Certainly, bioregulatory dentists utilize many treatments to neutralize these processes, the removal of galvanic currents and dental restoration treatment topping the list. In the short term, a powdered mineral therapy can alter the pH of saliva, helping to rewire a patient's "antenna" so to speak, decreasing their tissue sensitivity to these currents while also reducing the amount of mercury vapor emitted. Mercury fillings—neurotoxic, mineral displacing, galvanic current inducing—emit a vast array of bioregulatory disruptive actions. Next time you call your dentist's office, ask if they are still using mercury; if they are, it's time to find a new dentist (more on finding one and the benefits of bioregulatory dentistry in a minute). Now that we've covered the dangers of mercury amalgam fillings, the other toxic dental procedure we need to discuss is root canals.

Reconsidering Root Canals

A root canal is performed when the pulp, the living tissue inside of a tooth, becomes heavily inflamed and infected. If the infection goes untreated, it can cause pain or lead to an abscess. During a root canal procedure, the nerve and pulp are removed and the inside of the tooth pulp chamber is cleaned, disinfected, and sealed. The goal of a root canal, performed to avoid losing the tooth completely, is to eliminate the bacteria from the pulp chamber. To irradiate these bacteria—which likely initially showed up as a protective measure—a range of toxic antiseptic and antibacterial irrigating solutions, including sodium hypochlorite (NaOCl) and chlorhexidine (an antimicrobial), and combinations of antibiotics such as tetracycline and detergents such as MTAD are used.[11] It's like pulling a muddy buoy out of a dirty pond, cleaning it, then putting it back in the pond with the expectation that moss, mud, and other biofilms will not collect again.

These cleaning measures often do not stop bacterial reinvasion. Bacteria are everywhere, and they are commonly the first responders to any type of homeostatic disruption, especially in the mouth. Which is normally a good thing. The problem is that the type of bacteria that drop anchor in root-canaled teeth are often more deleterious than their predecessors, releasing potent toxins into the newly disinfected canal. And the root-canaled teeth no longer have a blood supply, so the bacteria inside root-canaled teeth are protected from the immune system. A root-canaled tooth is a dead tree limb still attached to a tree. A healthy tooth is a living, attached and bendable branch. Even the best root canal filling still leaves half of the organic space unfilled, and the bacteria invade. Root-canaled teeth can be a primary source of silent chronic infection and chronic, degenerative disease. The pathogenic bacteria found in these dead canals can travel to other sites in your body (especially if you are immunocompromised) and can potentially contribute to a number of different health problems, especially heart disease. Oral infections are the most common diseases of humankind and are also a key risk factor for heart disease, which is the leading cause of death worldwide.[12] The toxins found in the diseased myelin of multiple sclerosis patients are the same as those found in root-canaled teeth. When Dr. Weston Price conducted his extensive research into the destructive effects of root canals (detailed in his two-volume work *Dental Infections Oral and Systemic* and *Dental Infections and the Degenerative Diseases*), his conclusions, ignored by the orthodox dental establishment for over fifty years, generally suggest the removal of all root canals in a patient's mouth. This comes at a cost of thousands of dollars that few people can ever afford. While few of us question what happens in the dentist's office, it's time we did. In the conventional model, treatments and surgical procedures are largely working against our biology. Thankfully, you absolutely can achieve health if you have root-canaled teeth; it's a matter of identifying and addressing the bioregulating systems that might be reacting to them.

The Dangers of Nitrous Oxide

Ever had nitrous oxide? It's also called laughing gas, and it has been used in dentistry for over a hundred years. Its primary purpose is to reduce anxiety during invasive treatments, but what many people don't know is that the use of laughing gas irreversibly inactivates the active form of vitamin B_{12}, increasing levels of DNA damage, and it can cause cerebral atrophy, neurological issues, seizures, and apnea resulting in death. For those who know the methylation cycle and the impact of single nucleotide polymorphisms (SNPs), you know that vitamin B_{12} is required as a coenzyme for the methionine cycle. If you are one of the almost 50 percent of the population that has an MTHFR SNP (which can contribute to dysregulation in methylation, a key genetic process for silencing or activating certain genes), this means that you are at great risk for serious inflammation as a result of even a single instance of nitrous oxide use.

Introducing Bioregulatory Dentistry

A bioregulatory dentist doesn't just specialize in teeth, because for thousands of years, we've known that teeth are connected via meridians to the rest of the body. Every tooth has an organ connection, and because of this, an infection, inflammation—any disturbance—anywhere in the mouth will have a physiological impact elsewhere in the body. And the distant impact site is not happenstance. Most often, an infected tooth will create a systemic irritation along the meridian pathway it is connected to. The concept of meridians has been an integral part of TCM for thousands of years, providing the backbone of acupuncture. More recently, in the 1950s, a German physician, Dr. Reinhold Voll, developed a diagnostic schematic, assigning each tooth to a group of organs, joints, and glands. Voll demonstrated how electrical characteristics of an acupuncture meridian measurement point remote from an associated organ could reflect the pathology of the organ associated with the same meridian. For example, the front two middle teeth, called the incisors, are associated with the kidney and bladder. The lower bicuspids affect the intestinal system. Breasts are connected along the meridian of the upper first molars. Because of this, depending on which tooth is affected, the appropriate meridian—and associated organs—should also always be assessed and treated. So no, a bioregulatory dentist is not stuck in the mouth when they assess your teeth. They are looking at a global picture, and when there is a dental issue, they are considering how to treat it in the least invasive, most biocompatible way possible. Because of this, every bioregulatory dentist should be working alongside—or referring patients to—a bioregulatory physician.

Since 1984, the International Academy of Oral Medicine and Toxicology (IAOMT) has been a highly active organization for dentists, physicians, and allied researchers who consider biocompatibility to be their first concern. The IAOMT has created an extensive education and certification program that involves training in mercury, fluoride, the root canal issue, nutrition, detox, and infection/inflammation. This group makes it possible for current dental professionals to transition into a biological practice. Safe mercury amalgam removal therapy (SMART) certification ensures that a dentist has had proper training on how to safely remove mercury fillings. Safe for both the patient

and for the medical professionals who are performing the filling replacement. Sure, many dentists claim to be able to safely
remove mercury fillings, yet often the proper precautions are
not taken and the patient experiences the long-term effects of
mercury toxicity. Make sure you find a SMART-certified, bioregulatory dentist before ambling off down the road of cleaning
up your mouth.

To properly remove a mercury filling, all staff in a bioregulatory dentistry practice will wear protective gowns and properly
sealed respiratory masks. Old mercury fillings are removed with
super-strong suction, separated from the wastewater into an
isolated container, and then picked up by EPA-licensed agents.
Every removal of amalgam must be accompanied by a medicinal
elimination—specific supplements should be given prior to amalgam removal including vitamin C, while activated charcoal and
chlorella should be used during the procedure. And the detox
doesn't end after the toxic fillings are removed. Ideally, treatments
are individualized based on the patients' status (i.e., diet, epigenetics,
SNPs, detox capacity) and patients are followed—depending on
level of toxicity—for six months and up to two years (by both a
bioregulatory dentist and a bioregulatory physician), as mercury is
difficult to remove from the nervous system and the milieu. During
the procedure, the amalgam should be sectioned into chunks and
removed in pieces as large as possible. Copious amounts of water
to reduce heat and devices to capture mercury discharges should
also be used to reduce ambient mercury levels. Some bioregulatory
dentists might arrange for the patient to receive an IV with vitamin
C to help the body fight the stress of the procedure and alkaline
infusions that contain homeopathic formulations that support the
kidney and pituitary. Air filtration systems should be used, as should
dental dams. There is a lot that goes along with the safe removal of
mercury fillings. (For a full description of the SMART protocol
visit www.theSMARTchoice.com.) But once mercury amalgams
come out, what should go in?

For dental patients concerned about which mercury-free alternative to use as a filling material, some providers might recommend

a dental biocompatibility test, in which a patient's blood is evaluated for the presence of IgG and IgM antibodies to common chemical ingredients used in dental products. The patient is then provided with a detailed list of which name-brand dental materials are safe for their use and which ones could result in a reaction. (Two examples of labs that currently offer this service are Biocomp Laboratories and Clifford Consulting and Research.) Of course the comprehensive testing and treatment technologies used in bioregulatory medicine must extend into dentistry, and the two must work hand in hand—no more separation between the mouth and medicine. Oral evaluation goes well beyond the X-ray, and in fact, important biological disruptions such as inflammation of the jawbone do not even show up on X-rays! Rather, diagnostics such as thermography testing of the jaw and corresponding meridians, heavy-metal testing, dark-field microscopy of the living blood, CRT thermography, HRV, and subtle energy testing including electro-acupuncture and Vega bio-terrain analysis provide guidance to the treatment team for how to best optimize health. Cone beam computed tomography (CBCT) provides a three-dimensional panoramic X-ray, and can be performed using new digital technology allowing for significant reduction on patient's X-ray absorption levels.

Bioregulatory dentists fill cavities, clean teeth, and make bridges and implants. But concurrently, they are rooted in the concept that when treating teeth, they must consider the entire body—diet, lifestyle, and mental and emotional health. They also use technology that minimizes exposure to harmful chemicals. Why isn't this happening in every dental office? Why doesn't insurance routinely cover amalgam-filling removal? The reason is a ramshackle excuse—used widely in conventional medicine—that there is not enough scientific evidence of an improvement in health if mercury amalgams are removed. Of course, if mercury removal were mandated, there would be a massive escalation of health care costs and an increase in insurance premiums. The American Dental Association would have to admit that it had erred, an admission that could be met with massive lawsuits. So widespread removal is not happening. At least not yet. And finding safe oral health providers largely falls on the patient. Let's now consider a few at-home oral health considerations for you to swish around.

Preventive Oral Care at Home

The first—and most important—step to helping maintain oral health is to look at what is on your plate and in your glass. Avoiding sugar and fermentable carbohydrates is critical. Keeping added sugars below 30 grams per day for adults and 15 grams per day for children is the best place to start. Start counting your daily intake of sugar grams, including drinks such as fruit juices and sodas, and you'll likely be surprised at just how much you are consuming. Replace sugar with vegetables, wine with noncarbonated mineral water. As we've discussed, when we consume simple carbohydrates, like sugar and white flours, they ferment and produce acid that eats away at the enamel of our teeth and causes tooth decay. Constant consumption of simple fermentable carbohydrates leads to acid production that overwhelms the buffering capacity of saliva, and the oral pH balance shifts from alkaline to acidic.

To balance acidity, it's important to consume highly alkaline foods, including parsley, cucumber, kale, kelp, and other sea vegetables to maintain the acid balance in the mouth. Algae, both brown saltwater algae and green freshwater algae such as chlorella and spirulina, have the ability to bind heavy metals to their cellular surfaces and then be excreted in the stool. Consuming an algae-containing green drink once a day is almost as important as a good tooth brushing!

Phytic acid or phytate, found in edible seeds, grains (wheat, barley), legumes (black beans), and nuts, impairs the absorption of iron, zinc, and calcium. The amount of phytic acid in these foods can be reduced if you soak, sprout, or ferment them. Both your toothpaste and your mouthwash should also be considered part of your diet as they enter your body. Make sure you switch your oral care products to the brands mentioned earlier in this chapter.

The resurgence of an Ayurvedic medicine tradition called oil pulling has gained recent attention, but be careful, as it can have a detergentlike action. Swishing oils like coconut or sesame around in your mouth for ten to twenty minutes can help rebalance oral microbes, but it should *not* be done to excess. Use of a neti pot, a nasal passage cleaning technique and another Ayurvedic tradition, helps balance oral microbes and clear out inflammation and infection. In fact, use of a neti pot has been found to be highly effective at reducing symptoms of a sinus infection. Give it a try!

Throughout this book we've highlighted several diagnostics and treatments used in bioregulatory medicine. In the next chapter we go into a little more detail, treatment by treatment.

Introduction to Major Bioregulatory Medicine Diagnostic and Treatment Modalities

No matter how much it gets abused, the body can restore balance. The first rule is to stop interfering with nature.
—DEEPAK CHOPRA

The main reason for healing is love.
—PARACELSUS

The state-of-the-art testing and diagnostics used in bioregulatory medicine enable BioMed physicians and clinicians to identify the primary cause(s) of illnesses. BioMed practitioners integrate the results from dozens of different tests that go beyond the body's general physiology and evaluate structural integrity, biochemical individuality, nutritional deficiencies, epigenetic predispositions, regulatory and metabolic processes, energetic imbalances, and the individual's unique psycho-emotional history, such as losses and traumas, for example. Bioregulatory medical diagnostics take into account every element of the body, mind, energetics, metabolics, genetics, regulatory systems, and beyond. When it comes to what's inside a bioregulatory medicine physician's bag of treatments, you will find over one hundred different modalities utilized. In this reference chapter you will find a list of many these tests and treatments. Though far from exhaustive, this list provides an introduction and overview to the main bioregulatory assessments and treatments that might be foreign to allopathically versed readers.

The Assessments and Diagnostics in Bioregulatory Medicine

Dozens of different assessment, testing, and diagnostic procedures are used in bioregulatory medicine, including innovative technology from around the globe designed to not only detect the presence of disease, but also to assess its development from a milieu standpoint while preventing future ailments. Every bioregulatory system—every gland, cell, organ, and tissue, from immune to endocrine, cardiovascular to nervous—is connected and therefore must be assessed from both a prevention and a function standpoint. Testing methods include saliva, stool, serum, urine, temperature, and bioresonance testing. Where allopathic medicine relies on serum labs, radiation- or ultrasound-based imaging, and invasive scoping that shows pathology or disease after it is already present, the testing methods used in bioregulatory medicine allow for a noninvasive and nontoxic approach to early detection, prevention, and monitoring.

Bioimpedance Analysis (BIA)

A bioelectrical impedance analysis or bioimpedance analysis (BIA) is a simple, quick, child-friendly, and noninvasive technique used to measure body composition. We know that body composition (increased weight translates to increased disease risk) is directly related to health, and this test is an integral part of a health and nutrition assessment. BIA testing devices, for example the InBody Test, measure the changes in electrical current as it travels through body fluids and tissues to provide accurate analysis of intracellular water, extracellular water, total body water, dry lean mass, lean body mass, body fat mass, weight, skeletal muscle mass, body mass index, percent body fat, segmental lean analysis, segmental fat analysis, body composition history, and basal metabolic rate.

Blood (Serum) Chemistry Testing

A blood test is a laboratory analysis performed on a blood sample that is usually extracted from an arm vein via hypodermic needle or by finger prick. A complete blood count (CBC) and a comprehensive metabolic panel (CMP) provide a broad range of diagnostic information, including a person's metabolism, liver, kidney, or white and red blood cell status. These blood tests also measure the number, variety, percentage, concentration, and quality of platelets, red blood cells, and white blood cells, while also looking at glucose, electrolytes, and cholesterol. Various other important tests can be performed by looking at blood, including certain hormonal, inflammatory, and cancer markers. Annual blood testing is the primary detection method allopathic medicine uses to detect disease, however their broad range and geographical veritably of "normal" ranges limits the preventive aspect of their testing strategy. The way allopathic reference values are determined, approximately 95 percent of all blood tests are considered normal but far from optimal. When you get an annual checkup, there is only a 5 percent likelihood your conventional doctor will even mention there are any issues. In contrast, a bioregulatory physician will discuss your optimal values and explain how all the numbers are important in order to accurately and completely understand the metabolic imbalances that are present. Bioregulatory medicine providers view serum lab results with consideration given to the preventive range of a value, allowing for early detection of imbalances.

Cancer Profile (CA Profile)

Several different testing companies offer comprehensive panels that assesses hormone, antigen, and other cancer-specific markers, including carcinoembryonic antigen (CEA), that might provide early detection before cancer symptoms appear. While many cancers can take eight to ten or more years to develop, most will provide clues of their development, expressed in a tumor-coddling milieu, a milieu that has the ability to be altered if cancer cells are detected soon enough. Unfortunately though, allopathic palpation, X-ray, CT, MRI, PET, biopsy, and conventional tumor markers tend to reveal cancers that are already firmly established. Bioregulatory medicine is able to detect early patterns from these tests and use natural, nontoxic therapies to alter a cancer-promoting milieu before the disease is firmly established. We all have cancer cells that are normally kept in check by a healthy immune system, so immune system assessment is also important to properly determine the best treatment option, as the American Cancer Society estimates that one third of all cancers need no treatment.

Contact Regulation Thermography (CRT)

In this test, the temperature of the skin is taken in over one hundred different locations around the entire body, evaluating fifteen different organ systems. The bioregulatory medicine provider studies skin temperature patterns to determine the metabolic activity in the various parts of the body. The skin temperatures correspond to specific internal organs and tissues through viscerocutaneous reflexes and give data to the functionality of a person's present biological circumstances. Disturbances in the energy-conversion processes and reduced responses to the stress stimulus show up in the CRT thermographic scan as normal or hyperactive, degenerative or blocked. This is one of the most commonly used systemwide diagnostic tests in bioregulatory medicine.

Digestive Testing

Healthy digestion requires the presence of multiple enzymes, healthy bacteria, and the absence of parasites, infectious bacteria, and inflammatory metabolites; extensive blood, stool, and urine tests are commonly used to evaluate digestive function. Digestive function tests are used to uncover conditions including leaky gut, decreased pancreatic function, unbalanced digestive enzymes, dysbiosis (bacterial balance), inflammatory processes, celiac disease, allergies and sensitivities, hepatic detoxification blockages, and other bioindividual imbalances. The intestines contain the largest amount of lymphoid tissue in the body, known as GALT (gut-associated lymphatic tissue). Immune cells are produced within the GALT and this tissue is important in protecting the body from pathogens. With the rise of ADHD, ADD, autism, IBS, celiac disease, Crohn's disease, ulcerative colitis, migraines, chronic fatigue, fibromyalgia, and many other conditions, it is essential to evaluate the gastrointestinal system.

Digital Pulsewave Analysis (DPA)

With cardiovascular disease as the leading killer in America, a DPA test is an invaluable tool to assess arteriosclerosis and is also useful in evaluating the level of oxygen profusion to tissues. DPA is an FDA-approved device that is sensitive enough to pick up the earliest signs of cardiovascular disease and reduced blood circulation. It gives an accurate measure of the elasticity of a person's arteries and determines the biological age of arteries. It provides information regarding mean heart rate, missed heartbeats (arrhythmias), level of arterial stiffness, arterial elasticity, remaining blood volume, the waveform of heart rate variability, the balance of the autonomic nervous system, and more. All this data is gleaned through a painless detector placed over the finger.

Electrodermal Testing

Electrodermal testing has been used successfully in Europe since 1953, originating with the German electro-acupuncture technique as developed by Dr. Reinhold Voll. This is a specialized noninvasive form of electrical resonance testing that is used to identify possible cellular imbalances or stressors that might be affecting the body's electrical system, including sensitivities to food, fats, sugars, alcohol, chemicals, and also is used to detect patterns of asthma, hay fever, skin problems, hormonal imbalances, and psycho-immunologic conditions. This painless procedure involves measuring potential differences (voltage) between a tip electrode held against an acupuncture point and a large surface electrode (hand electrode) held by the patient. The resultant resistance is then measured.

Food Allergy and Sensitivity Testing

It is estimated by some groups that more than 60 percent of the global population cannot digest certain protein molecules in commonly consumed foods, including wheat and milk. A 2011 study in the journal *Pediatrics* found that 30 percent of children have multiple food allergies.[1] Symptoms are many and can include: diarrhea, indigestion, nausea, passing excessive amounts of gas, vomiting, itching, and nasal congestion. Knowing what foods are triggering symptoms *and* the inherent associated immune response is a very important element of bioregulatory medicine. Two of the antibodies involved in allergic reactions are immunoglobulin E (IgE) and immunoglobulin G (IgG). IgE production occurs right after ingestion or inhalation of an allergen and is referred to as a Type I immediate hypersensitivity reaction. In contrast, IgG antibodies are produced several hours or days after exposure to an allergen and are called Type III, or delayed hypersensitivity reactions. Allergy serum test assays detect both immediate and delayed reaction to allergens through IgE and IgG respectively. Food sensitivities can be tested via various energetic and blood tests and also with a mediator release test (MRT), which measures the immune and inflammatory responses to both foods and synthetic food-chemicals.

Heavy-Metal and Environmental Toxin Assessment

Heavy metals and environment toxins, such as volatile solvents, polychlorinated biphenyls (PCBs), phthalates, parabens, chlorinated pesticides, organophosphates, and bisphenol A, all need to be evaluated and eliminated in order to optimize health. Toxins, as we've learned, can bind to and block hormone function while also causing a plethora of symptoms including headaches, fatigue, weight gain, and muscle and joint pain. Toxins are the biggest source of bioregulatory blockages. In today's toxic world, many people have elevated levels of toxins that contribute to inflammation, autoimmune disease, and poor health. The presence of heavy metals and environmental toxins can be attained through hair analysis, blood testing, and urine testing. Assessment of heavy metals and toxic burden is a standard of care in bioregulatory medicine.

Heart Rate Variability Test (HRV)

The heart rate variability (HRV) test is a quick electrophysiology study assessing the stress on a person's autonomic nervous system (ANS). The test evaluates heart rate variability when at rest and gives an assessment of the adaptability of the sympathetic and parasympathetic branches of the ANS. To achieve health and balance, the body needs to maintain a proper balance between the sympathetic, "fight or flight" nerves and the parasympathetic "rest and digest" nerves, which is increasingly difficult due to the daily demands of the world. The HRV test can detect early signs of the development of pathological processes or the presence of some functional disorders that might not be revealed by an ordinary physical examination. (This test was detailed in chapter 6.)

Hormone Analysis

A hormone analysis allows us to assess the levels of these powerful chemical messengers that alter the way that distant cells and tissues work. Hormones are essential for bodily functions, metabolic activity, and brain function. Small amounts of hormone are secreted by glands into the bloodstream to deliver profound effects on metabolism in other areas of the body. It is vital to evaluate adrenal, gonadal (testes/ovaries), thyroid, and pituitary glands together to effectively get a complete picture and to identify the root cause of hormonal dysfunction. Evaluation of hormones can be done through saliva, blood, and urine testing, as appropriate. One of the newest modalities in modern medicine is the field called Age Management Medicine. From this perspective, we look at all of the hormone levels in a patient and make interventions to normalize the hormones that are deficient or elevated. Hormone testing helps the bioregulatory medicine provider to properly address common hormone imbalances including menopause, thyroid imbalance, and infertility, among others. When it comes to hormone imbalance, the bioregulatory goal is to also find and eliminate the underlying causes of aberrant hormone levels so that the patient takes the least amount of medications as possible over the long term.

Genetic Testing

Various genetic tests are designed to measure how your body processes medications, hormones, food, and more. Different people metabolize biologically active substances differently. Some people process medications too quickly, too slowly, or not at all. Understanding how your genes affect your reaction to certain substances can help reduce adverse effects, especially those caused by drugs. These tests can also identify alternative medications that are better suited for you based on your genetic profile. In addition, identifying genetic SNPs can help the bioregulatory medicine provider fine-tune nutrition and supplemental protocols in order to circumvent under- or over-functioning genes. Genetic tests are generally very easy to complete and can be done in a provider's office or in the privacy of your own home. A simple cheek swab test or blood sample can collect all the DNA needed for this once-in-a-lifetime test.

Neuroscan

This type of brain imaging and mapping is designed to assist the understanding of the electrophysiological functioning of the brain. These tests can provide high-density electroencephalogram recordings, electromagnetic source localization, multimodal neuroimaging, and enhancements to functional MRI. A neuroscan is a type of neurodiagnostic test that is performed when a patient's illness or condition is thought to be based in the central nervous system (brain and spinal cord). It can be used for anything from mental health issues to diagnosing brain tumors.

Nutrient Testing

Assessing and identifying levels of vitamins, antioxidants, minerals, trace minerals, and amino acids is a very important way to identify the presence of either deficiencies or excess that can contribute to physical and mental health, and also to a disease process. Practically every physiological function in the human body requires nutrients for proper function. Vitamin and mineral compounds play a key role in immune system modulation and fortification, inhibiting inflammation, protecting against free radical damage, and maintaining hormonal balance including insulin, thyroid, reproductive hormones, adrenal hormones, and neurotransmitters. As the Environmental Working Group found, almost 93 percent of the American population is deficient in at least one nutrient.[2] Nutrient levels can be assessed through urine and blood and sometimes in hair.

Parasitology and Pathogen Screening

A parasitology and pathogen screening evaluates the presence of parasites, beneficial bacteria, imbalanced gut flora, pathogenic bacteria, and yeast. These tests can help reveal the often masked causes of acute or chronic conditions that might stem from parasitic infection or an impaired or imbalanced gut microbiome. The parasite evaluations used in bioregulatory medicine are much more extensive than the allopathic stool tests that look for only four or five different pathogens and are usually only run in cases of acute gastrointestinal conditions such as diarrhea. In addition, assessing the presence of chronic viral infections including Lyme, Epstein-Barr, and cytomegalovirus is very important, as they are linked to chronic and degenerative illness. Parasitology and pathogen testing can be done using blood or stool.

Vega (Bioresonance)

Vega testing is the culmination of decades of German electroacupuncture testing development and is a synthesis between Chinese medical knowledge and cutting-edge Western technology. It is an energetic regulatory technique that records the bioelectric potential of a person and is capable of revealing functional or so-called energetic disorders. This painless process consists of measuring potential differences (voltage) between a tip electrode held against an acupuncture point and a large surface electrode (hand electrode) held by the patient. The resultant resistance is then measured. The electro-conductivity of the point might signify degenerative disease within an organ, systemic inflammation, or more specific imbalances including various infections, yeast overgrowth, and presence of heavy metals, among other things.

Zyto Scan

This nontoxic, painless, and noninvasive testing method uses a proprietary system that correlates energetic signatures or impulses with physical substances including foods, supplements, vitamins, or body systems and organs and environmental factors such as parasites and toxins. The computer signatures resulting from this correlation are called virtual stimulus items. A Zyto biocommunication scan introduces subtle energetic impulses of over one hundred virtual stimulus items to the body through the use of a hand cradle. The body then emits a natural response to this communication and the Zyto software records the responses. There are different types of bioscans (also called biosurveys); some biosurveys are general in nature while others focus specifically on organs in the body or on environmental factors like toxins and allergens.

Biotherapies and Treatment Technologies

Biotherapies are treatments intended to stimulate or restore homeostasis to the body's many bioregulating systems. Natural, noninvasive, and nontoxic, the therapeutics used in bioregulatory medicine embody the Hippocratic principle of "First do no harm." Therapeutic skill is a science, an art, and a creative process. The therapeutic modalities of bioregulatory medicine, like its diagnostics, are as individual and varied as the creative processes signature to the practitioners who use them. The therapies of bioregulatory medicine extend beyond the conventional treatment of disorders of structure and function with a one-gene-one-target approach, to encompass energetic imbalances, disorders of regulation and adaptation, and social and psycho-emotional disturbances and themes. Various therapies might be delivered intravenously, subcutaneously, orally, physically, via a nebulizer, or via electrical energetics. The therapeutic practices of bioregulatory medicine also largely nod to the mind-body paradigm. Here we introduce some of the more commonly used therapies in bioregulatory medicine. For a complete list, visit www.brmi.online/therapeutics. Bioregulatory medicine practitioners individualize treatment options based on intake and diagnostics. Patients decide their treatments with their practitioner and follow with a certain self-responsibility. Bioregulatory medicine can only be the guide and companion; the patients are in the driver's seat and it becomes their responsibility to apply any at-home treatments with discipline and reliability.

Acupuncture

Acupuncture, a three-thousand-year-old healing technique of traditional Chinese medicine, literally means "to puncture with a needle in a strategic site." During these treatments, needles are used alone or in combination with another modality called moxibustion. *Moxibustion* is the burning on or over the skin of selected herbs. Scientific studies coupled with thousands of years of anecdotal evidence have confirmed the effectiveness of acupuncture in treating many conditions, including chronic pain; headaches; menstrual cramps; low back, neck, or muscle pain; osteoarthritis; spastic colon; depression; and anxiety. Acupuncture also can improve the functioning of the immune system while helping to reduce side effects from conventional treatments, including chemotherapy.

Anthroposophical Medicine

Anthroposophical medicine was founded nearly a hundred years ago by Dr. Rudolf Steiner and Dr. Ita Wegman. It is an integrative multimodal treatment system based on a holistic understanding of man and nature and of disease and treatment. Anthroposophical medicine utilizes medicines derived from plants, minerals, and animals, while also using art therapy, eurythmy therapy, rhythmical massage, counseling, and psychotherapy. It is established in eighty countries worldwide, most significantly in Central Europe. Over two hundred clinical studies on the efficacy of anthroposophic medicine have shown positive outcomes and high tolerability.

Antihomotoxic Therapy

This medical modality and therapy was developed by German physician Dr. Hans-Heinrich Reckeweg, who also founded the company Heel and its flagship remedy, Traumeel, which contains thirteen different homeopathic remedies at single potencies, and is one of the top-selling homeopathic remedies in the world. The aim of antihomotoxic medicine lies in the activation of self-cure powers of the organism with weak stimuli. It is similar to homeopathy, but the focus is on bioregulating systems that are blocked due to the presence of homotoxins. Antihomotoxicology introduces an additional toxin similar to the present disruptive substance that is potentized in accordance with official homeopathic pharmacopeia and is intended as a stimulus for the body to elicit a healing and restorative activation, stimulation, and regulation. These therapies and formulas are varied based on a person's phase of disease.

BioMat

The BioMat is a state-of-the-art, FDA-approved medical device that delivers therapeutic far infrared rays, negative ions, and the conductive properties of amethyst channels to help relieve pain, improve immune function, and reduce stress. Far infrared rays are part of the electromagnetic light spectrum and are close to the light frequency of natural sunlight. An ion is a particle containing an electrical charge. An ion with a negative electrical charge is called a negative ion, and this type of ion is now considered to be integral to healthy cellular function. Use of a BioMat stimulates ion channels by producing negative ions that deliver energy to the cells of the body. The anecdotal healing properties of amethyst have been acknowledged and celebrated for centuries by ancient scientists and healers due to the highly conductive properties of this mineral. Amethyst crystals offer the most consistent and powerful delivery of far infrared light waves and ionic effects to the human body. A noninvasive and relaxing treatment, use of this specific therapeutic device requires nothing more than sitting or lying atop the mat for a designated period of time.

Biomodulation and Bioresonance

Biomodulation, also known as biofeedback, bioresonance, or resopathy, is the reactive or associative adjustment of a patient's biochemical or cellular status. The principles of bioresonance therapy are used in electrodermal testing, biophysical information therapy (BIT), bioenergetic therapy, energy medicine, and vibrational medicine. These treatments encompass the regulation of innate electrophysiological, chemical, and molecular pathways through relatively low-intensity physical and chemical interventions including microcurrents, lasers, and nonpharmaceutical substances. The various treatment devices that fall under the umbrella of biomodulation are noninvasive and state-of-the-art, powered by proprietary software and high-performance microchip processors. They provide effective symptomatic relief and management of chronic pain, as well as conditions such as fatigue, allergies, digestive disorders, and insomnia.

Chelation Therapies

Chelation is the binding of metals (such as mercury, arsenic, lead, and cadmium), or minerals (such as calcium), to a substance considered the "chelator." The Greek word *chele* means "to claw." Initially, the medical use of chelating agents was to treat heavy-metal poisonings. The chelating agent ethylene diamine tetraacetic acid (EDTA), a synthetic amino acid, was first introduced into medicine in the United States in 1948 as a treatment for lead poisoning incurred by workers in a battery factory. Other chelation agents used in bioregulatory medicine to remove heavy metals and other xenobiotics include dimercaptosuccinic acid (DMSA or succimer) and dimercaptopropane sulfonate (DMPS). Chelation treatments are typically carried out over several weeks or months via IV therapy or oral medication and must be closely monitored by a bioregulatory physician or dentist well versed in chelation therapy and patient assessment.

Colon Hydrotherapy

This treatment is essential to any detoxification program and is vital in preventive programs to optimize health and wellness. It removes wastes, fermentation, and toxins from the liver, intestines, and colon while also providing hydration and oxygenation to these organs and tissues. A step up from a home enema, in colon hydrotherapy an experienced hydrotherapist will insert a sterile tube into the rectum and slowly infuse water or other substances, including coffee and probiotics, into that cavity. This procedure stimulates the liver to produce more bile, thus moving out old, sluggish, toxin-laden bile into the small intestine for elimination. Colon hydrotherapy also stimulates the production of glutathione-S-transferase, an enzyme used by the liver to make the detox pathways run efficiently. The increase in glutathione, one of the main conjugation chemicals, enables toxins to be eliminated via bile into the small intestines while also minimizing the backlog of yet-to-be-detoxified biological and environmental toxins. A key therapy when it comes to drainage and detoxification, various forms of colon hydrotherapy have been used across every medical model for thousands of years.

Craniosacral Therapy (CST)

Osteopathic physician Dr. William Sutherland developed the modality of craniosacral therapy (CST) in the 1930s. This approach targets the craniosacral system, which includes the structures of the central nervous system including the skull, cranial sutures, cerebrospinal fluid, membranes of the brain, and the vertebrae, spinal cord, and sacrum. The craniosacral system is highly interconnected with the musculoskeletal system, the vascular system, and the sympathetic and parasympathetic nervous systems. Trauma anywhere in the body might impact the craniosacral system, restricting normal movement and creating regulatory blockages. CST uses a series of gentle techniques to remove these blocks and restore the subtle movement, or pulse, in the central nervous system. CST uses extremely light finger pressure and does not involve the manipulation or chiropractic "adjustment" of the skeletal system.

Electromagnetic Field (EMF) Therapy

This treatment modality uses electromagnetic frequencies or pulses to stimulate metabolic healing, support detoxification, improve lymphatic flow, increase microcirculation, improve cellular membrane integrity, stimulate cellular regeneration, and decrease inflammation, while also benefiting chronic musculoskeletal issues, broken bones, chronic fatigue, fibromyalgia, and nervous system and digestive disorders. Used for over one hundred years, EMF therapy gained international recognition during the Soviet space explorations, when pulsed electromagnetic field therapy (PEMF) was used by the cosmonauts to help reduce the loss of bone density that occurs when people are removed from the Earth's gravitational and magnetic fields. Various FDA-approved devices are used today.

Electrical Muscle Stimulation

Electrical muscle stimulation, also known as neuromuscular electrical stimulation (NMES) or electromyostimulation, is the elicitation of muscle contraction by using electric impulses. EMS has proven

to be a successful and noninvasive tool, particularly in sports medicine, for strength training and post-exercise recovery. It has also
proven to be successful as a rehabilitation and preventive tool for
partially or totally immobilized patients. The impulses are generated
by a device and are delivered through electrodes on the skin near
to the muscles being stimulated. The electrodes are generally pads
that adhere to the skin. The impulses mimic the action potential
that comes from the central nervous system, causing the muscles to
contract, and this contraction provides a stimulus for healing.

Flower Essences

Flower essences are dilute extracts of various types of flowers and
plants that are useful in management of all health problems. They are
similar to homeopathic remedies in that they are diluted and potentized to make them more effective than just using the original flower
as an herbal extract. The original thirty-eight flower remedies were
developed by Dr. Edward Bach (1886–1936), an English physician
and homeopathic practitioner who devoted the last years of his life
to researching and developing his remedies. Dr. Bach believed that all
diseases of the body come about as a result of imbalances or negativity
at the level of the soul, and by correcting the problem there, healing
would result and the body would be able to heal on all levels. The
flower remedies, which are mild-tasting liquid drops taken orally, act
to balance harmonies in the emotional and spiritual body, and bring
about a gentle healing by bringing the body back in balance with
itself. In this way, they are able to help even functional and physical
problems. Rescue Remedy is one example of a flower essence that is
very helpful in both humans and pets during times of acute anxiety.
Today there are many companies throughout the world that manufacture flower essences; they have expanded the scope and power of these
remedies beyond the original thirty-eight discovered by Dr. Bach.

Gemmotherapy

Gemmotherapy is a branch of phytotherapy (more specifically
embryo-phytotherapy) that was discovered by Pol Henry, a Belgian
physician and homeopath. It has been further detailed and developed

into a clinical application by Dr. Max Tetau. Dr. Henry proposed the idea of using the embryonic parts of plants in phytotherapy as a potentially more effective means of drainage. In fact, it was homeopathic drainage principles that inspired Dr. Henry to investigate the possibility of capturing the vitality of the plants by preparing macerates from fresh embryonic tissue. These tissues possess different properties than herbal extracts made from other parts of the plant or the same plant once it has matured. More specifically, they are rich in growth factors, including phytohormones, auxins (a hormone found in plants), and gibberellins. Auxins have a fetal hormonal action and are found only in the buds of a plant. Gibberellins stimulate RNA and protein synthesis, and like the auxins, they are present only in the buds of the plant. They have a rejuvenating effect on the tissues and organs for which they have an elective affinity known as organotropic.

Herbal Medicine

Herbal medicine, also called botanical medicine or phytomedicine, refers to using a plant's seeds, berries, roots, leaves, bark, or flowers for medicinal purposes. Herbalism has a long tradition of use outside conventional medicine. Chinese herbal medicine is one of the great herbal systems of the world, with an unbroken tradition going back to the third century BC. Plants and natural substances are used for therapy or medicinal purposes to treat many conditions, such as allergies, asthma, eczema, premenstrual syndrome, rheumatoid arthritis, fibromyalgia, migraine, menopausal symptoms, chronic fatigue, irritable bowel syndrome, and cancer, among others. Commonly used herbs include: echinacea (*Echinacea purpurea* and related species), St. John's wort (*Hypericum perforatum*), and milk thistle (*Silybum marianum*). These herbs can be taken orally via liquid or in capsule form, or also as teas or applied topically.

Homeopathic Medicine

Homeopathy is a medical modality created in 1796 by the German physician Samuel Hahnemann, and is based on the age-old doctrine of like cures like (*similia similibus curentur*). Homeopathic remedies, of which there are now over three thousand, are naturally occurring substances (plant, animal, or mineral) that would cause the symptoms of a disease in healthy people but are intended to cure similar symptoms in sick people. The selection of a homeopathic agent is strictly suited to the individual. Worldwide, over two hundred million people use homeopathy on a regular basis. Homeopathy is included in the national health systems in a number of countries, including Brazil, Germany, Belgium, France, Chile, India, Mexico, Pakistan, Switzerland, and the United Kingdom. Homeopathic medicine has shown great success in treating a vast array of acute and chronic physical disorders and diseases and also emotional imbalances. These nontoxic formulas are also safe and effective remedies for children. For example, arnica (mountain daisy) is the leading remedy in sports medicine and first aid, used for injury-related shock and trauma. It also helps to reduce pain from injury and to speed the healing process. On an emotional front, ignatia (St. Ignatius bean) is one of the leading homeopathic medicines for acute grief, anxiety, and depression, especially after a death or separation from a loved one. Despite a 2017 FDA statement against the validity of homeopathics, they continue to be one of the safest and most effective therapies used worldwide.

Hyperthermia

Hyperthermia is one of the most powerful immune-stimulating treatments, and is therefore highly anticancer, antiviral, and antibacterial, yet it is underutilized and largely unknown in North America. Hyperthermia treatment involves raising the temperature of either the whole body or a localized area to 39–43°C (102–109°F). Research has shown that high temperatures stimulate cellular immunity and can damage cancer cells, usually with minimal injury to normal tissues. The immune system's defense cells work best at a temperature above 39°C (102°F). At that temperature, all metabolic and detoxification processes are intensely stimulated. The body often naturally creates a fever during acute illness, and this rise in temperature helps overcome infections, inflammations, and pain much quicker and more effectively. Hyperthermia has significant systemic and localized biological effects. It helps to combat aging;

supports detoxification, cardiovascular health, athletic performance, immune enhancement, and circulation; and improves metabolic and endocrine function. It can decrease lactic acid and circulating CO_2 while facilitating cellular waste removal. In Europe, hyperthermia is often utilized as an adjunctive therapy with various conventional cancer treatments, such as chemotherapy and radiotherapy, while in other clinics it is used alongside biological regulatory therapies.

Immunotherapies

Bioregulatory medicine uses various natural substances to help stimulate and direct the immune system in acute, chronic, and degenerative disease processes. Bioregulatory medical providers use dozens of medicinal mushrooms, such as the immune-system-strengthening lion's mane (*Hericium erinaceus*), which has a long history in TCM. Mistletoe (*Viscum album*), also known as *Iscador*, Helixor, or Isorel in European countries, is another immunotherapy agent used by bioregulatory medicine practitioners. In European countries, mistletoe is regarded as an effective medication for treating cancer. Mistletoe extract has been shown to kill cancer cells in laboratory animals and to boost the immune system by increasing the number of white blood cells, and it is classified as a biological response modifier and as anti-angiogenic. Natural thymic peptides are used by bioregulatory medicine practitioners not only to enhance immune system functioning but also to act as transmitters between the neuroendocrine and immune systems.

IV Therapy

Various types of bioregulatory therapies are best administered intravenously (IV). For example, nutritional formulas (a Myers' cocktail) and antioxidants such as glutathione are used for the treatment of a wide range of clinical conditions and also to enhance performance and recovery in professional athletes. Vitamin C and mistletoe are also given via IV. When nutrients are given intravenously, they bypass the digestive system in order for a much higher level of nutrition to be delivered directly to your cells through the bloodstream. The nutrients then feed those cells that are sluggish, help provide an immediate therapeutic response by correcting deficiencies that might arise due to biological imbalances, and support the detoxification process.

Lymphatic Drainage Treatments

All of the various manual or machine-assisted lymphatic treatments, including physical vibration with sonic or acoustic waves and electropressure, are extremely low in energy and are gentle and safe. These treatments improve edemas, fibrotic conditions, and swollen lymph nodes, helping to treat inflammation, chronic pain, joint aches, allergies, sinus issues, respiratory problems, headaches, prostate problems, hormone imbalance and chronic female conditions, dental traumas and chronic problems, heavy-metal toxicity, neuromuscular trauma, and immune and fatigue syndromes. The lymphatic system transports and cleanses every cell and organ in the body. It is the pathway for toxins to be removed from the body and, because white blood cells are transported through lymph, it plays a key role in immune function. Lymphatic treatments help to remove congestion, allowing more nutrients to be supplied to the cells, removing toxins, and increasing immune function.

Neural Therapy

Neural therapy is based on the concept that trauma can produce long-standing disturbances in the electrochemical function of tissues and a local disturbance might cause symptoms in unrelated and distal sites. Scars and scar tissue are considered to be very significant interference fields. Scar tissue has a different membrane potential than normal cells, and when a cell has lost its normal membrane potential, the ion pumps in the cell wall stop working and abnormal minerals and toxic substances accumulate inside the cell. As a result, the cell loses its ability to heal itself and resume normal functioning. Neural therapy corrects the disturbance in the tissue by reestablishing the normal electrical conductivity of cells via therapeutic local anesthetic. One common combination anesthetic is Traumeel and procaine injected into trigger points and rigid muscles. While Traumeel is anti-inflammatory, stimulates tissue healing, and has an analgesic action, procaine acts on the cell wall to allow the ion pumps to resume normal action and restore the membrane potential, correcting the bioelectric disturbance at a specific site or nerve ganglion. By reestablishing the normal electrical conductivity of cells and nerves, the disturbed functions are also restored to normal, and the patient returns to health as far as this is anatomically still possible. Intended goals include pain alleviation and antihistamine and antihyperergic effects, and those with chronic pain, orthopedic disorders, circulation disorders, and more can benefit from this form of therapy.

Neurofeedback

Neurofeedback, also called neurotherapy or neurobiofeedback, is a type of biofeedback that uses real-time displays of brain activity—most commonly electroencephalography—to teach self-regulation of brain function. Biofeedback therapy helps reduce a wide range of physical symptoms by lowering sympathetic activation and provides a noninvasive, effective psychophysiological intervention for psychiatric disorders. It is a mind-body technique in which individuals learn how to modify their physiology for the purpose of improving physical, mental, emotional, and spiritual health, and has been used to treat common disorders including anxiety, autism, depression, eating disorders, high blood pressure, muscle pain or tension, anxiety, IBS symptoms, insomnia, and schizophrenia. (Neurofeedback is described in more detail in chapter 6.)

Nosode Therapy

Constantine Hering (1800–80), the "father of homeopathy in the United States," created nosode therapy. A nosode is a potentiated dose of a disease in question; taking a nosode for a specific germ boosts immunity and confers a level of protection from contracting it. For example, the nosode for flu prevention is oscillococcinum, the nosode for diptheria is diptherinum, the nosode for tuberculosis is tuberculinum, and the one for measles is morbillinum. Nosodes can be made from any pathological material derived from plant, animal, or human sources. They are gaining traction in the treatment of Lyme disease and also as alternatives to vaccination.

Nutrition, Nutraceutical Therapy, and Orthomolecular Medicine
Nutrients are the building blocks of life and are required for normal physiological and emotional function. Bioregulatory medicine focuses on the assessment of nutrient deficiencies, food allergies, and sensitivities in order to bioindividualize a therapeutic diet (e.g., ketogenic or seed cycling) and nutraceutical plan. The term *nutraceutical* combines *nutrient* (a substance that provides nourishment for growth or metabolism) and *pharmaceutical* (a medical drug). A nutraceutical thus represents a product that contains food-derived nutrients and is often concentrated in liquid, capsule, powder, or pill form.

Orthomolecular medicine, established by Linus Pauling in 1968, is the restoration and maintenance of health through the administration of adequate amounts of substances that are normally present in the body, including vitamins, minerals, trace elements, essential fatty acids, amino acids, flavonoids, herbs, and accessory food factors.

Oligotherapy

Oligotherapy, developed by French physician Dr. Jacques Ménétrier, uses small concentrations of minerals as opposed to the more common macrodoses frequently used in nutritional supplements. Minerals are a fundamental component of nearly every biological enzyme reaction, and oligotherapy is a unique way to affect the enzymatic process. French chemist Gabriel Bertrand used the word *oligo* (small) to describe the enzymatic cofactors that are essential in biochemical reactions. Oligotherapy uses mineral elements in concentrations that are exactly equal to the level required for enzymatic activity. The distribution of these elements in an ionic solution (approximately equal to a 12X dilution) allows them to be absorbed directly into the bloodstream (sublingually), and to be used immediately for catalytic activity, either stabilizing or activating enzymes. While oligotherapy is not truly homeopathic, the doses used are certainly capable of acting on an energetic level.

Organotherapy

Organotherapy, or biological mRNA therapy, is used to restore homeostasis to diseased organs, glands, and tissues by means of replacement via animal glandular and tissue extracts that are diluted and dynamized

according to homeopathic principles. UNDA organotherapy remedies, for example, are prepared from porcine, sheep, and rabbit sources
that are specially raised for therapeutic use. Pituitary extracts from pigs,
for instance, can be used to treat hormone disorders. One of the pillars
of bioregulatory medicine—drainage and detoxification—calls upon
diluted and dynamized organ tissues to stimulate corresponding organ
tissues. Organotherapy products typically contain elements, trace elements, amino acids, lipids, and so forth in a biologically quantitative
and organically compatible relationship to the associative human
organs. There are several different classifications of organothera-
peutic remedies, including tissue preparations, extracts from cells
(immune cells, osteoblasts), and microbial therapeutic remedies.

Oxygen Therapies

There are many factors that contribute to oxygen loss in the body,
such as internal and external pollutants, mental strain, physical
overstrain, disease, and trauma. In addition, as we age, our bodies
become less effective at delivering oxygen to our cells, increasing
the chances of degeneration and disease. Oxygen is the most critical
nutrient we consume. Nothing is as consistent and as predictable
as the gradual, linear decline in oxygen utilization seen in all aging
populations. Aging and the diseases of aging are caused primarily
by decreased oxygen utilization. This decrease leads to the excessive
free radical production that results in degenerative disease. Thus,
various different oxygen therapies help increase oxygen in the
cells, where it helps convert nutrients into usable ATP required
to create energy. One such oxygen therapy is called exercise with
oxygen therapy, or EWOT, and is a therapy of choice for professional athletes. Breathing concentrated oxygen while exercising can
provide an immediate increase in strength, endurance, and energy
by increasing the level of oxygen in the blood, plasma, and tissues.
When used to treat chronic and degenerative diseases, EWOT
significantly increases plasma oxygen levels, aids in detoxification,
decreases tissue hypoxia, flushes lactic acid, and improves circulation.
    Hyperbaric oxygen therapy (HBOT) is a long-used treatment for
the decompression sickness that can occur when scuba divers rise to

the surface too quickly. The body's natural healing processes are significantly enhanced by inhalation of 100 percent oxygen, and over the years, many other conditions have also been found to respond to HBOT. Treatments can be done in a special type of room called a hyperbaric oxygen chamber, where a person is completely immersed in 100 percent oxygen that is delivered at high pressure. They can also be given through a gas mask, which delivers 100 percent oxygen directly to the lungs. HBOT can treat various conditions, including wounds that aren't healing in response to conventional treatment, carbon monoxide poising, some brain and sinus infections, burns, and bone infections, and it is recently gaining attention for a cancer treatment.

Ionized oxygen therapy (IOT) has been utilized and researched since the 1920s, with most of the work being done in Germany. It is intended to mimic nature where singlet oxygen is formed on the surface of the leaves of plants and trees through a process called photosensitization. Photosensitization requires oxygen, light, and a proper photosensitizer, like chlorophyll, which can act like a catalyst to transfer the light energy to the oxygen. The result is singlet oxygen, with a distinctively high level of energy. IOT devices, such as the Valkion, convert normal air into singlet oxygen and provide a powerful reduction in free radicals, aid detoxification, increase energy production, and reduce cholesterol, triglycerides, uric acid, and overall inflammation.

Ozone Therapy

Along the same vein as oxygen therapies, ozone (O_3) is a gas discovered in the mid-nineteenth century and is a molecule consisting of three atoms of oxygen. Ozone therapy has been utilized and heavily studied for more than a century. In 1896 Nikola Tesla patented the first O_3 generator in the United States. Its effects are proven, consistent, and safe and convey minimal and preventable side effects.[3] Medical O_3 is able to inactivate bacteria, viruses, fungi, yeast, and protozoa, to stimulate oxygen metabolism, and to activate the immune system. It conveys many health benefits, especially in the dental field in treating cavities, and has also been found to decrease blood cholesterol and stimulate antioxidative responses. Ozone therapy is being used to treat aging, cancer, and autoimmune disorders such as systemic lupus erythematosus, rheumatoid arthritis, and multiple sclerosis. Ozone therapy can be administered multiple ways including through IV, rectally, nasally, vaginally, and into the ear canal.

Phytotherapy

Closely related to herbal medicine, phytotherapy is the intended medical use of plants and plant extracts for therapeutic purposes. This plant therapy consists of using potent plant remedies made from fresh buds and young shoots of growing plants. Macerated in water, natural glycerin, and alcohol, they are standardized to a 1:20 extract to ensure delivery of concentrated active extracts to targeted organs. In Germany, phytotherapy is classified as a regular discipline of orthodox science-oriented medicine and has been beneficial in the treatment of chronic inflammatory diseases of the digestive tract, including gastritis, Crohn's disease, ulcerative colitis, rheumatoid arthritis, ankylosing spondylitis, psoriasis, scleroderma, dermatitis, psoriasis, diabetes, and atherosclerosis.

Psychosomatic Bodywork (PSB)

PSB therapy encompasses a wide range of modalities that explore the mind-body connection. It incorporates elements of physiotherapy, osteopathy, chiropractic, shiatsu, Rolfing, bioenergetics, visceral manipulation, lymphatic drainage massage, biofeedback, craniosacral therapy, polarity therapy, and kinesiology. It is used to detect and release both acute and chronic structural resistances, and helps to treat skeletal misalignments, muscular spasms, fascial restrictions, neural entrapments, poor joint mobility, spasms of visceral organs, stagnation of lymph, cerebrospinal fluid or venous stasis, as well as bioenergetic blockages. Because structural resistances are the somatic equivalents of unprocessed traumatic experiences, PSB can also precipitate psychotherapeutic healing.

Sauna

Saunas and sweat lodges have been used across the globe for thousands of years. Because sweating and increased body temperature activate many of the same physiological responses as physical exercise, sauna bathing has historically been used as a proven method to stimulate bodily detoxification, but is also regarded as a type of physical training, and so today it is commonly used among athletes. During a thirty- to forty-five minute sauna session, the adult body can burn about three hundred calories as the heart rate increases to about twice its resting rate and the sympathetic nervous system and hypothalamic-pituitary-adrenal axis are intensely activated to compensate for the excessive increase of body temperature. Some studies suggest that regular sauna bathing might lower the blood pressure in patients with hypertension while also promoting relaxation of the muscles and a release of toxins and other impurities through the pores that are opened via heat treatment.[4] Sauna has also shown efficacy in treating skin problems and respiratory issues, and lowering risk of dementia and Alzheimer's. Some bioregulatory medical clinics have infrared saunas, a type of sauna that uses light to create heat. This type of sauna is sometimes called a far infrared sauna—*far* describes where the infrared waves fall on the light spectrum. Where a traditional sauna uses heat to warm the air, an infrared sauna heats your body directly without warming the air around you.

Sound and Other Sensory-Targeted Therapies

Bioregulatory medicine regularly harnesses the energetic medical powers of light, color, sound, and vibration—for example through harmonic sound translation, audio-color (Vega), primordial sounds, Vedic sound therapy, signature sound works, vibrational healing, tuning forks, soundbed therapy, and various bioresonance therapies. These energetic therapies affect the nervous system, conveying positive effects to heart rate, respiration, brain waves, and mood. One example, sound, when played in harmony, will move water molecules into a visible pattern, a phenomenon known as resonance. Our bodies are 60 percent water and cells are largely made of water, and the water inside us transmits the sound and vibrations that can encourage a state of relaxation. These types of therapies, nontoxic and side-effect-free, have been shown to decrease pain, anxiety, and sleep disorders.

Tissue (Cell) Salts

Tissue salts were developed in the 1870s by Wilhelm Heinrich Schussler, a German biochemist, physicist, and homeopathic doctor. Dr. Schussler conducted research demonstrating that, when reduced to ashes, each human cell contains twelve minerals or biochemic tissue salts that occur naturally in our bodies and all organic matter on Earth, such as plants, rocks, and soil. Thus, these minerals should be present in all living cells in perfect balance to ensure good health. Imbalance, or a deficiency of any of the tissue salts, causes disease, and the body begins to develop symptoms associated with the tissue salts that are lacking. Restoring the correct balance of tissue salts in the body will therefore help to remove the symptoms and restore health and vitality. In varying combinations these tissue salts exist in every cell in your body. The twelve tissue salts are: Calcarea fluorica, Calcarea phosphorica, Calcarea sulphurica, Ferrum phosphoricum, Kalium muriaticum, Kalium phosphoricum, Kalium sulphuricum, Magnesium phosphoricum, Natrium muriaticum, Natrium phosphoricum, Natrium sulphuricum, and Silicea. Tissue salts work effectively in conjunction with other forms of healing; they address imbalance on a cellular level.

Unani Medicine

Unani medicine is a system of complex homeopathic remedies that are synergistically formulated with plant constituents to target and carry potentized metals to specific organs where enzymatic and metabolic functions are carried out on a cellular level, helping to enhance the body's innate ability to remove toxins from the system. These combination homeopathic drainage remedies are composed of substances that have traditionally been used for specific organs or tissues. For example, remedies for the liver (*Chelidonium*, *Taraxacum*), kidney (*Berberis*, *Solidago*), skin (*Saponaria*, *Viola tricolor*), and lung (*Euphrasia*, *Sabadilla*, *Verbascum*) are often prescribed to help stimulate drainage in those detoxification and emunctory organs.

Bioregulatory Organizations and Clinics

O ver the last fifty years, several organizations have been founded for the promotion of biological regulatory medicine. The world is now blessed with a few excellent organizations, societies, and institutes that foster bioregulatory medicine. The following listing is not complete, but it might serve as a pathfinder.

The Biological Medicine Network

http://www.marioninstitute.org/programs/biomed-network

The Biological Medicine Network, the leader in bringing bioregulatory medicine to the United States, was founded to disseminate information on biological regulatory medicine. Part of their network includes annual conferences, training and certification programs, and the flagship clinic, the American Center for Bioregulatory Medicine and Dentistry (ACBMD), which is the largest and most complete biological medicine clinic in North America, one that incorporates both biological medicine and dentistry together in a state-of-the-art facility. The sister clinic, the American Center for Biological Medicine, is located in Scottsdale, Arizona. The nonprofit arm of the BioMed Network is the Bioregulatory Medicine Institute (BRMI), founded to promote the science and art of biological regulatory medicine and to increase public knowledge of bioregulatory medicine as a holistic and evidence-based medical system.

Congress for Biological Medicine, Baden Baden

http://www.medwoche.de

Since 1966, the Congress for Biological Medicine, also known as Medizinische Woche Baden-Baden, has been conducting conferences on biological regulatory medicine in Baden Baden, Germany. Located in the beautiful resort town of Baden Baden, the congress is a unique showcase for the many therapeutic and diagnostic innovations that are part of biological regulatory medicine. More than four thousand doctors of all fields, dentists, medical students, and several hundred exhibitors attend the congress annually.

The Canadian Society of Bioregulatory Medicine (CSBRM)

http://www.csbrm.ca

The CSBRM is an independent and inclusive medical society that promotes homotoxicology, homeopathy, and bioregulatory medicine. It is a national organization created for the purpose of enhancing the knowledge and acceptance of bioregulatory medicine throughout Canada.

Occidental Institute Research Foundation

http://www.oirf.com

In 1972 in Canada, the Occidental Institute Research Foundation was founded as an information and technology bridge linking top German practitioners and suppliers involved in aspects of German biological medicine with progressive English-speaking practitioners around the world.

International Academy of Biological Dentistry and Medicine (IABDM)

https://iabdm.org

The IABDM is a network of dentists, physicians, and allied health professionals committed to caring for the whole person—body, mind, spirit, and mouth. They are dedicated to advancing excellence in the art and science of biological dentistry, and they encourage the highest standards of ethical conduct and responsible patient care.

The International Academy of
Oral Medicine and Toxicology (IAOMT)

https://iaomt.org

The IAOMT is a nonprofit organization dedicated to protecting public health and the environment since it was founded in 1984. It is dedicated to seeking the safest, least toxic way to accomplish the goals of modern dentistry, and is a leader in informing consumers about health risks from mercury amalgams ("silver fillings") and water fluoridation.

The International Society for Bioregulatory Medicine (ISBM)

http://bioregmed.com

Founded in London in 1972, the ISBM is an international board-certified specialist body, pioneering the cause for bioregulatory medicine. The society formalizes training standards and competencies for its affiliates worldwide.

US BioMed Centers

The American Center for Bioregulatory Medicine and Dentistry of New England

111 Chestnut Street
Providence, Rhode Island 02903
833-8BIOMED (phone)
http://www.biomedcenterne.com

The American Center for Biological Medicine

9312 E. Raintree Drive
Scottsdale, Arizona 85260
888-982-2260 (phone)
http://www.thebiomedcenter.com

The goal of providing access to European bioregulatory medicine in the United States has been a direct response to more than twenty years of public demand. A massive wave of medical service consumers have not only recognized but also insisted that each individual needs to be treated as a unique matrix of interconnectedness—physically, mentally, emotionally, and spiritually—and that their nontoxic medical treatment plans need to be tailored accordingly. While many patients have traveled to Europe for this type of care, there has been an increasing demand to have clinics in North America. As a result, there are currently two comprehensive and collaborative BioMed centers located in North America—one on each coast. The American Center for Biological Medicine (ACBM), a bioregulatory medical treatment and training facility, is located in Scottsdale, Arizona. It was founded in 2011 by Dr. Jeoffrey Drobot, NMD (http://www.drdrobot.com), and Dr. Dickson Thom, DDS, ND, who both continue as the clinics' medical directors. As the outpouring of unparalleled clinical results from bioregulatory medicine have continued to quickly spread, an East Coast facility became essential. Thus, the end result of a Marion Institute (an innovative social-change and nonprofit organization) incubation project is the flagship, 12,770-square-foot Bioregulatory Medical and Dental Clinic of New England (the BioMed Center) that opened in 2018 in Providence, Rhode Island.

Both state-of-the-art BioMed facilities offer a sweeping range of diagnostic and therapeutic technologies designed to promote the body's intrinsic mechanisms for self-regulation and self-healing. Personalized, whole-body wellness is the focus at all current and future BioMed Centers, where patients experience a unique blend of traditional and modern technologically advanced diagnostics and treatments. Treatment modalities include energy medicine, hyperthermia, pulsed magnetic field therapy, lymphatic therapies, IV therapy, immunotherapy, structural and message therapy, ozone therapy, colon hydrotherapy, and chelation detoxification, among others. The East Coast BioMed Center has the largest bioregulatory dental clinic in North America, directed by Dr. Gerald Curatola, DDS, author of the groundbreaking book

The Mouth-Body Connection. Detoxification, education, advanced treatments, detailed and focused follow-up care, and healing are all part of every BioMed patient experience, whether they come for an annual prevention exam, chronic and degenerative illness treatments, or performance enhancement.

There are many internship, education, training, and certification programs offered and being developed nationwide as part of the Bioregulatory Medicine Network (BioMed Network), which can be found at https://www.marioninstitute.org/programs /biomed-network. Another arm of the BioMed Network includes the Bioregulatory Medicine Institute (BRMI), directed by Dr. James Odell, ND, OMD, L.Ac., which holds biannual conferences and has a free informational website for those looking to learn more about bioregulatory medicine or link to books, articles, podcasts, and newsletters: https://www.brmi.online. BioMed clinics and programs are overseen by a medical advisory board, including Switzerland-based Concièrge Medical Services provider Dr. Frank Pleus (http://www.dr-pleus.com), and staffed by expert and leading-edge medical physicians and professionals. All BioMed clinics are designed and equipped for those looking for a new prevention and primary care model, to treat chronic or degenerative illness, or to optimize health and performance. BioMed clinics and providers look beyond short-term symptom treatment, and rather support patients of all ages throughout a lifelong health and healing journey.

NOTES

Introduction: Patient-Focused Medicine

1. Samuel Hahnemann, *Organon of Medicine* (Los Angeles: J. P. Tharcher, 1982).
2. Martin A. Makary and Michael Daniel, "Medical Error—the Third Leading Cause of Death in the US," *BMJ* 353 (2016): i2139, doi:10.1136/bmj.i2139.

Chapter One:
Modern Disease and the Rise of the Allopathic Model

1. Douglas C. Wallace, "A Mitochondrial Paradigm of Metabolic and Degenerative Diseases, Aging, and Cancer: A Dawn for Evolutionary Medicine," *Annual Review of Genetics* 39 (2005): 359.
2. Steve R. Pieczenik and John Neustadt, "Mitochondrial Dysfunction and Molecular Pathways of Disease," *Experimental and Molecular Pathology* 83, no. 1 (2007): 84–92, doi:10.1016/j.yexmp.2006.09.008.
3. J. Neustadt and S. R. Pieczenik, "Medication-Induced Mitochondrial Damage and Disease," *Molecular Nutrition and Food Research* 52 (2008): 780–88, doi:10.1002/mnfr.200700075.
4. "Medicine Use and Spending in the U.S.," IQVIA, May 4, 2017, https://www.iqvia.com/institute/reports/medicines-use-and -spending-in-the-us-a-review-of-2016.
5. James Raftery and Maria Chorozoglou, "Possible Net Harms of Breast Cancer Screening: Updated Modelling of Forrest Report," *BMJ* 343 (2011): d7627, doi:10.1136/bmj.d7627.
6. Mahyar Etminan, Mohsen Sadatsafavi, Siavash Jafari, Mimi Doyle-Waters, Kevin Aminzadeh, and J. Mark FitzGerald, "Acetaminophen Use and the Risk of Asthma in Children and Adults: A Systematic Review and Metaanalysis," *CHEST* 136, no. 5 (2009): 1316–23, doi:10.1378/chest.09-0865.
7. Shelly L. Gray, Melissa L. Anderson, Sascha Dublin, Joseph T. Hanlon, Rebecca Hubbard, Rod Walker, Onchee Yu, Paul K. Crane, and

Eric B. Larson, "Cumulative Use of Strong Anticholinergics and Incident Dementia: A Prospective Cohort Study," *JAMA Internal Medicine* 175, no. 3 (2015): 401–7, doi:10.1001/jamainternmed .2014.7663.

8. J. A. McDougall et al., "Long-Term Statin Use and Risk of Ductal and Lobular Breast Cancer among Women 55 to 74 Years of Age," *Cancer Epidemiology, Biomarkers, and Prevention* 22, no. 9 (2013): 1529–37, doi:10.1158/1055-9965.EPI-13-0414.

9. Preetha Anand, Ajaikumar B. Kunnumakara, Chitra Sundaram, Kuzhuvelil B. Harikumar, Sheeja T. Tharakan, Oiki S. Lai, Bokyung Sung, and Bharat B. Aggarwal, "Cancer Is a Preventable Disease That Requires Major Lifestyle Changes," *Pharmaceutical Research* 25, no. 9 (2008): 2097–2116, doi:10.1007/s11095-008 -9661-9.

10. Martin A. Makary, Heidi N. Overton, and Peiqi Wang, "Overprescribing Is Major Contributor to Opioid Crisis," *BMJ* 359 (2017): j4792, doi:10.1136/bmj.j4792.

11. Ciddi Veeresham, "Natural Products Derived from Plants as a Source of Drugs," *Journal of Advanced Pharmaceutical Technology & Research* 3, no. 4 (2012): 200–1.

12. Charles Ornstein, Mike Tigas, and Ryann Grochowski Jones, "Now There's Proof: Docs Who Get Company Cash Tend to Prescribe More Brand-Name Meds," *ProPublica*, March 17, 2016, https:// www.propublica.org/article/doctors-who-take-company-cash-tend -to-prescribe-more-brand-name-drugs.

13. Martin A. Makery and Michael Daniel, "Medical Error—the Third Leading Cause of Death in the US," *BMJ* 353 (2016): i2139, doi:10.1136/bmj.i2139.

14. Biljana Bauer Petrovska, "Historical Review of Medicinal Plants' Usage," *Pharmacognosy Reviews* 6, no. 11 (2012): 1–5.

15. "Emotions and Disease," NIH US National Library of Medicine, https://www.nlm.nih.gov/exhibition/emotions/index.html.

16. Hans Selye, *The Stress of Life* (New York: McGraw-Hill, 1984).

17. T. N. Bonner, *Iconoclast: Abraham Flexner and a Life in Learning* (Baltimore: Johns Hopkins University, 2002).

18. Beverly Rubik et al., "Biofield Science and Healing: History, Terminology, and Concepts," *Global Advances in Health and Medicine* 4 (2015): 8–14.

19. Rubik et al., "Biofield Science and Healing."

Chapter Two:
Bioregulatory Medicine: The Future of Health and Healing

1. S. Acosta et al., "NT-020, a Natural Therapeutic Approach to Optimize Spatial Memory Performance and Increase Neural Progenitor Cell Proliferation and Decrease Inflammation in the Aged Rat," *Rejuvenation Research* 13, no. 5 (2010): 581–88.

Chapter Three:
Implementing a Systems-Based Approach to Bioregulation, Regeneration, and Healing

1. M. C. Brum, F. F. Filho, C. C. Schnorr, G. B. Bottega, and T. C. Rodrigues, "Shift Work and Its Association with Metabolic Disorders," *Diabetology & Metabolic Syndrome* 7, no. 1 (2015): 1.

2. Robert K. Navaiux, "Metabolic Features of the Cell Danger Response," *Mitochondrion* 16 (2014): 7–17, doi:10.1016/j.mito.2013.08.006.

3. Mark P. Mattson et al., "Meal Frequency and Timing in Health and Disease," *Proceedings of the National Academy of Sciences of the United States of America* 111, no. 47 (2014): 16647–53.

4. University of Alabama at Birmingham Public Relations, "Time-Restricted Feeding Study Shows Promise in Helping People Shed Body Fat," *ScienceDaily*, January 6, 2017, https://www.sciencedaily.com/releases/2017/01/170106113820.htm.

5. W. Osler, "The Study of the Fevers of the South," *JAMA* XXVI (1986): 1001–4. https://www.ncbi.nlm.nih.gov/pmc/articles/PMC4056101/#B1.

6. A. Ghezzi and M. Zaffaroni, "Neurological Manifestations of Gastrointestinal Disorders, with Particular Reference to the Differential Diagnosis of Multiple Sclerosis," *Neurological Sciences* 22, supplement no. 2 (2001): S117–22.

Chapter Four:
Detoxification: Homotoxicology and Biotherapeutic Drainage

1. Alastair Crisp, Chiara Boschetti, Malcolm Perry, Alan Tunnacliffe, and Gos Micklem, "Expression of Multiple Horizontally Acquired Genes Is a Hallmark of Both Vertebrate and Invertebrate Genomes," *Genome Biology* 16, no. 1 (2015): 50, doi:10.1186/s13059-015-0607-3.

2. Cui-Cui Liu, Hao Yang, Ling-Ling Zhang, Qian Zhang, Bo Chen, and Yi Wang, "Biotoxins for Cancer Therapy," *Asian Pacific Journal of Cancer Prevention* 15, no. 12 (2014): 4753–58.

3. Hussein I. Adbel-Shafy and Mona S. M. Mansour, "A Review on Polycyclic Aromatic Hydrocarbons: Source, Environmental Impact, Effect on Human Health and Remediation," *Egyptian Journal of Petroleum* 25, no. 1 (2016): 107–23, doi:10.1016/j.ejpe.2015.03.011.

4. "How Much Is Too Much?: Appendix B: Vitamin and Mineral Deficiencies in the US," EWG, June 19, 2014, https://www.ewg.org/research/how-much-is-too-much/appendix-b-vitamin-and-mineral-deficiencies-us.

5. Wendee Holtcamp, "Obesogens: An Environmental Link to Obesity," *Environmental Health Perspectives* 120, no. 2 (2012): a62–a68.

6. Roberta F. White et al., "Recent Research on Gulf War Illness and Other Health Problems in Veterans of the 1991 Gulf War: Effects of Toxicant Exposures during Deployment," *Cortex* 74, supplement C (2016): 449–75, doi:10.1016/j.cortex.2015.08.022.

7. Christopher A. Taylor, "Deaths from Alzheimer's Disease—United States, 1999–2014," *Morbidity and Mortality Weekly Report* 66, no. 20 (2017): 521–26, doi:10.15585/mmwr.mm6620a1.

8. "Infertility," National Center for Health Statistics, Centers for Disease Control and Prevention, https://www.cdc.gov/nchs/fastats/infertility.htm.

9. "Western Sperm Counts 'Halved' in Last 40 Years," PubMed Health, July 26, 2017, https://www.ncbi.nlm.nih.gov/pubmedhealth/behindtheheadlines/news/2017-07-26-western-sperm-counts-halved-in-last-40-years.

10. "How High-Tech Baby Making Fuels the Infertility Market Boom," *Time Money*, July 9, 2014, http://time.com/money/2955345/high-tech-baby-making-is-fueling-a-market-boom.

Chapter Five:
Diet: Digestion, Nutrition, and Plant Medicine

1. Briana Pobiner, "Evidence for Meat-Eating by Early Humans," *Nature Education Knowledge* 4, no. 6 (2013): 1.

2. Tamara Bhandari, "Popular Heartburn Drugs Linked to Higher Death Risk," Washington University School of Medicine in St. Louis, July 3, 2017, https://medicine.wustl.edu/news/popular-heartburn-drugs-linked-higher-death-risk.

3. K. Ryan Wessells and Kenneth H. Brown, "Estimating the Global Prevalence of Zinc Deficiency: Results Based on Zinc Availability in National Food Supplies and the Prevalence of Stunting," *PLoS ONE* 7, no. 11 (2012): e50568.

4. Michael Janson, "Orthomolecular Medicine: The Therapeutic Use of Dietary Supplements for Anti-Aging," *Clinical Interventions in Aging* 1, no. 3 (2006): 261–65.

5. K. Pallav et al., "Noncoeliac Enteropathy: The Differential Diagnosis of Villous Atrophy in Contemporary Clinical Practice," *Alimentary Pharmacology & Therapeutics* 35, no. 3 (2012): 380–90.

6. B. Lonnerdal, "Dietary Factors Influencing Zinc Absorption," *Journal of Nutrition* 130 (2000): 1378S–85S.

7. Donald R. Davis, Melvin D. Epp, and Hugh D. Riordan, "Changes in USDA Food Composition Data for 43 Garden Crops, 1950 to 1999," *Journal of the American College of Nutrition* 23, no. 6 (2004): 669–82.

8. Mike Amaranthus and Bruce Allyn, "Healthy Soil Microbes, Healthy People," *The Atlantic*, June 11, 2013, https://www.theatlantic.com /health/archive/2013/06/healthy-soil-microbes-healthy -people/276710.

9. B. B. Petrovska, "Historical Review of Medicinal Plants' Usage," *Pharmacognosy Reviews* 6, no. 11 (2012):1–5, doi:10.4103/0973 -7847.95849.

10. Keith I. Block et al., "Designing a Broad-Spectrum Integrative Approach for Cancer Prevention and Treatment," *Seminars in Cancer Biology* 35, supplement (2015): S276–S304, doi:10.1016/j.semcancer .2015.09.007.

11. James Odell, "Mistletoe Therapy," Bioregulatory Medicine Institute, September 28, 2017, https://www.brmi.online/single-post/2017/09 /28/Mistletoe-Therapy.

Chapter Six:
The Nervous System: Reuniting the Mind with Medicine

1. "2015 Stress in America," American Psychological Association, March 10, 2016, http://www.apa.org/news/press/releases/stress/2015 /snapshot.aspx.

2. "Nearly 7 in 10 Americans Take Prescription Drugs, Mayo Clinic, Olmsted Medical Center Find," Mayo Clinic, June 19, 2013, https:// newsnetwork.mayoclinic.org/discussion/nearly-7-in-10-americans -take-prescription-drugs-mayo-clinic-olmsted-medical-center-find.

3. Tatiana Falcone, "Childhood Emotional Trauma Closely Linked to Problems in Adulthood," Cleveland Clinic, November 6, 2014, https://consultqd.clevelandclinic.org/2014/11/childhood-emotional -trauma-closely-linked-to-problems-in-adulthood; and Shakira F.

Suglia et al., "Childhood and Adolescent Adversity and Cardiomet-abolic Outcomes: A Scientific Statement from the American Heart Association," *Circulation* 137 (2018): e15–e28, doi:10.1161/CIR.0000000000000536.

4. "Humor Helps Your Heart? How?," American Heart Association, April 5, 2017, http://www.heart.org/HEARTORG/HealthyLiving/Humor-helps-your-heart-How_UCM_447039_Article.jsp.

5. Mak Adam Daulatzai, "Non-Celiac Gluten Sensitivity Triggers Gut Dysbiosis, Neuroinflammation, Gut-Brain Axis Dysfunction, and Vulnerability for Dementia," *CNS & Neurological Disorders Drug Targets* 14, no. 1 (2015): 110–31.

6. H. Shalev, Y. Serlin, and A. Friedman, "Breaching the Blood-Brain Barrier as a Gate to Psychiatric Disorder," *Cardiovascular Psychiatry and Neurology* (2009): 278531, doi:10.1155/2009/278531.

7. S. N. González-Díaz, A. Arias-Cruz, B. Elizondo-Villarreal, and O. P. Monge-Ortega, "Psychoneuroimmunoendocrinology: Clinical Implications," *The World Allergy Organization Journal* 10, no. 1 (2017): 19, doi:10.1186/s40413-017-0151-6.

8. S. S. Virani et al., "Takotsubo Cardiomyopathy, or Broken Heart Syndrome," *Texas Heart Institute Journal* 34 (2007): 76–79.

9. B. Weinhold, "Epigenetics: The Science of Change," *Environmental Health Perspectives* 114, no. 3 (2006): A160–67.

10. Sara Reardon, "Poverty Linked to Epigenetic Changes and Mental Illness," *Nature News*, May 25, 2016, doi:10.1038/nature.2016.19972.

11. S. T. Y. Azeemi and S. M. Raza, "A Critical Analysis of Chromotherapy and Its Scientific Evolution," *Evidence-based Complementary and Alternative Medicine* 2, no. 4 (2005): 481–88, doi:10.1093/ecam/neh137.

12. Yoshihisa Koike, Mitsuyo Hoshitani, Yukie Tabata, Kazuhiko Seki, Reiko Nishimura, and Yoshio Kano, "Effects of Vibroacoustic Therapy on Elderly Nursing Home Residents with Depression," *Journal of Physical Therapy Science* 24, no. 3 (2012): 91–294, doi:10.1589/jpts.24.291.

13. J. M. Randall, R. T. Matthews, and M. A. Stiles, "Resonant Frequencies of Standing Humans," *Ergonomics* 40, no. 9 (1997): 879–86, doi:10.1080/001401397187711.

14. "Shattering Cancer with Resonant Frequencies," Gateway for Cancer Research, October 21, 2015, https://www.gatewaycr.org/gateway-blog/posts/2015/october/shattering-cancer-with-resonant-frequencies.

Chapter Seven:
The Mouth of Medicine: Mercury, Toothpaste Toxins, and the Oral Microbiome

1. J. Kim and S. Amar, "Periodontal Disease and Systemic Conditions: A Bidirectional Relationship," *Odontology* 94, no. 1 (2006): 10–21, doi:10.1007/s10266-006-0060-6.

2. Y. W. Han, "Fusobacterium Nucleatum: A Commensal-Turned Pathogen," *Current Opinion in Microbiology* 0 (2015): 141–47, doi:10.1016/j.mib.2014.11.013.

3. S. Shweta and S. K. Prakash, "Dental Abscess: A Microbiological Review," *Dental Research Journal* 10, no. 5 (2013): 585–91.

4. Michael Gröschl, "The Physiological Role of Hormones in Saliva," *BioEssays* 31, no. 8 (2009): 843–52, doi:10.1002/bies.200900013.

5. J. Li et al., "The Tonsil Microbiome Is Involved in Rheumatoid Arthritis," *Annals of the Rheumatic Diseases* 76 (2017): 509.

6. M. Kilian et al., "The Oral Microbiome: An Update for Oral Healthcare Professionals," *British Dental Journal* 221, no. 10 (2016): 657–66, doi:10.1038/sj.bdj.2016.865.

7. P. Grandjean and P. J. Landrigan, "Neurobehavioural Effects of Developmental Toxicity," *The Lancet Neurology* 13, no. 3 (2014): 330–38, doi:10.1016/S1474-4422(13)70278-3.

8. Alessia Carocci, Nicola Rovito, Maria Stefania Sinicropi, and Giuseppe Genchi, "Mercury Toxicity and Neurodegenerative Effects," *Reviews of Environmental Contamination and Toxicology* 229 (2014): 1–18, doi:10.1007/978-3-319-03777-6_1..

9. R. Dufault et al., "Mercury Exposure, Nutritional Deficiencies and Metabolic Disruptions May Affect Learning in Children," *Behavioral and Brain Functions* 5 (2009): 44, doi:10.1186/1744 -9081-5-44.

10. Ghazal Mortazavi and S. M. J. Mortazavi, "Increased Mercury Release from Dental Amalgam Restorations after Exposure to Electromagnetic Fields as a Potential Hazard for Hypersensitive People and Pregnant Women," *Reviews on Environmental Health* 30, no. 4 (2015): 287–92, doi:10.1515/reveh-2015-0017.

11. Z. Fedorowicz, M. Nasser, Byron P. Sequeira, R. F. de Souza, B. Carter, and M. Heft, "Irrigants for Non-surgical Root Canal Treatment in Mature Permanent Teeth," *Cochrane Database of Systematic Reviews* 8 (2012): CD008948, doi:10.1002/14651858 .CD008948.pub2.

12. Karim El Kholy, Robert J. Genco, and Thomas E. Van Dyke, "Oral Infections and Cardiovascular Disease," *Trends in Endocrinology & Metabolism* 26, no. 6 (2015): 315–21, doi:10.1016/j.tem .2015.03.001.

Chapter Eight:
Introduction to Major Bioregulatory
Medicine Diagnostic and Treatment Modalities

1. Ruchi S. Gupta, Elizabeth E. Springston, Manoj R. Warrier, Bridget Smith, Rajesh Kumar, Jacqueline Pongracic, and Jane L. Holl, "The Prevalence, Severity, and Distribution of Childhood Food Allergy in the United States," *Pediatrics* (June 2011), peds.2011-0204, doi:10.1542/peds.2011-0204.

2. Environmental Working Group, "Appendix B: Vitamin and Mineral Deficiencies in the US," in *How Much Is Too Much?: Excess Vitamins and Minerals in Food Can Harm Kids' Health* (Washington, DC: Environmental Working Group, accessed January 8, 2018), https:// www.ewg.org/research/how-much-is-too-much/appendix -b-vitamin-and-mineral-deficiencies-us#.WzTrgakpBBw.

3. Masaru Sagai and Velio Bocci, "Mechanisms of Action Involved in Ozone Therapy: Is Healing Induced Via a Mild Oxidarive Stress?," *Medical Gas Research* 1, no. 29 (2011), doi:10.1186/2045-9912-1-29.

4. Francesco Zaccardi et al, "Sauna Bathing and Incident Hypertension: A Prospective Cohort Study," *American Journal of Hypertension* 30, no. 11 (November 2017): 1120–25, doi:10.1093/ajh/hpx102.

INDEX

AbM (*Agaricus blazei* Murill), 124–25
absorption of nutrients
    leaky gut effects on, 113
    overview, 110–11
    phytates effect on, 113
    in the small intestine, 112
acid-alkaline balance
    bioregulatory remedies for
        restoring, 121
    role in homeostasis, 117–120
    in the urine, 72
acid deposits, 119
acid-forming foods, reducing
    consumption of, 120
acid reflux, 118
acquired immunity, 68
acupoint stimulation techniques, 146
acupuncture, 145–46, 186–87
acute toxic exposures, potential
    reversibility of, 86–87
addiction, to psychopharmaceuticals,
    19, 130
addictive effects, as term, 19
adenosine triphosphate (ATP), 14
adrenaline, increase in with stress, 133, 135
adrenal phase, 54
adverse effects, as term, 19
Agaricus blazei Murill (AbM), 124–25
Age Management Medicine, 183
agriculture practices, loss of nutrients
    from, 115
algae, consumption of, 175
alkaline foods, increasing consumption
    of, 120, 175
alkaloids
    medical benefits of, 125–26
    overview, 123
allergies and sensitivities, food, 113–14,
    181–82
allopathic medicine
    attempts to utilize bioregulatory
        medicine, 6
    deaths related to, 20

development of pharmacology, 23–25
focus on pharmaceuticals, 11, 17–21
impact of discovery of DNA, 32–33
modern diseases, 13–16, 33–34
origin of term, 23
origins of medical theories and
    philosophies, 21–23
quantum theory and energy
    medicine, 29–32
recent naturopathic focus on, 8–9
rise of empiricism, 25–29
suppression of symptoms vs. healing,
    17–21
use of specialists, 74
views on health, 16–17
alpha brain waves, 140
Alzheimer's disease
    increasing rates of death from, 90
    phytochemical treatments for, 38
    symptom similarity to mercury
        poisoning, 168
amalgam fillings. *See* fillings, dental
American Center for Biological
    Medicine, 203, 205–7
American Center for Bioregulatory
    Medicine and Dentistry of New
    England, 203, 205–7
American Chemical Society, 29
American College of Cardiology, 63
American Dental Association, 156,
    167, 174
American Heart Association, 63
*American Journal of Respiratory and Critical
    Care Medicine*, 18
amethysts, healing properties of, 188
AMP-activated protein kinase
    (AMPK), 52
Anatomy of the Spirit (Myss), 151
animal protein, balanced consumption
    of, 119–120
anthroposophical medicine, 46, 187
antibiotic resistance, 117
antibiotics, overuse of, 116–17

antibodies
acquired immunity and, 68
autoimmune disorders and, 89
immunoglobulins, 112, 174, 182
in the intestines, 112
antihistamines, long-term use concerns, 18
antihomotoxic therapy, 97–99, 187–88
antinutrients, in processed foods, 103
antioxidants, 77, 122, 123
Apigenin, 38
apothecaries, development of, 24
arnica (mountain daisy), 193
atherosclerosis, 62
athletic performance. *See* sports medicine
and performance
ATP (adenosine triphosphate), 14
atrazine, 85–86
autoimmune disorders
bioregulatory approach to, 69
rise in, 68, 89, 115
role of toxins in, 88–89
autonomic nervous system
heart rate variability testing of, 17, 63,
136–37, 182–83
overview, 71, 134
auxins, 192
Ayurveda
constitutional typing in, 148
neti pots, 176
oil pulling, 175
origins of, 21–22
seasonal herbal cleansings, 93

Bach, Edward, 191
Bachmann, F., 43
back pain, emotional factors in, 133
Bacon, Francis, 26
bacteria
dietary concerns, 115–17
gut microbiome, 114–17, 185
oral microbiome, 156, 158, 160–61,
162–64
root canal concerns, 170–71
bad breath (halitosis), 163
Beauchamp, Antoine, 27
Bernard, Claude, 40
Bertrand, Gabriel, 197
beta-glucans, immune system benefits, 124
BIA (bioimpedance analysis), 178
Bifidobacterium spp., 116

Biocomp Laboratories, 174
biocycles, 49–50, 79
biofeedback (biomodulation), 139–140,
188–89
See also neurofeedback
biofields, 31, 137–140
bio-hacking, as term, 43
bioimpedance analysis (BIA), 178
Biological Medicine Network, 203, 207
Biological Medicine Society, 43
biological mRNA therapy (organotherapy),
197–98
biological remedies and therapies, 186–202
acupuncture, 145–46, 186–87
anthroposophical medicine, 46, 187
antihomotoxic therapy, 97–99, 187–88
BioMat device, 188
biomodulation (biofeedback), 139–140,
188–89
biopharmaceuticals vs., 6
biotherapeutic drainage principles, 97–99
chelation therapy, 99, 189
chiropractic medicine, 70
colon hydrotherapy, 189–190
color therapy, 142–43, 201
craniosacral therapy, 190
electrical muscle stimulation, 190–91
electromagnetic field (EMF) therapy, 190
energetic therapies, 141–44, 201
flower essences, 191
focus on curing vs. suppressing
symptoms, 10–11
gemmotherapy, 191–92
herbal medicine, 192
homeopathic medicine overview, 97–98,
192–93
hyperthermia, 193–94
immunotherapies, 194
individualized treatment plans, 9–10,
126–27, 186
intravenous (IV) therapy, 195
lymphatic drainage treatments, 67–68, 195
neural therapy, 195–96
neurofeedback, 71–72, 140–41, 151, 196
nosode therapy, 196
nutritional therapies, 197
oligotherapy, 197
ongoing evaluation and adjustment of, 10
organotherapy, 197–98
orthomolecular medicine, 110, 121, 197

ABOUT THE AUTHORS

Dr. Dickson Thom, DDS, ND, one of the cofounders and medical directors of the American Center of Biological Medicine, has over forty years of experience as a clinician and over twenty years as a medical professor. He lectures extensively throughout North America and is the author of *Coping with Food Intolerances* and *Unda Numbers: An Energetic Journey to Homeostasis and Wellness.* Dr. Thom has been teaching doctors, students, and the lay public on proven medical principles and business skills for over thirty-five years. His first postdoctoral degree was obtained from the Faculty of Dentistry, University of Toronto, in 1974. He then received his degree in naturopathic medicine from the Canadian College of Naturopathic Medicine in 1986. In 1989 he completed a second degree from the National University of Naturopathic Medicine (NUNM) in Portland, Oregon. Dr. Thom was the dean of naturopathic medicine at NUNM and a full-time professor teaching clinical and physical diagnosis, gastroenterology, X-ray practicum, neurology, and business entrepreneurship for twenty-three years.

In 2009 Dr. Thom received the prestigious Vis Award from the American Association of Naturopathic Physicians for his commitment to the Vis or "Healing Power of Nature." In addition to being a full-time professor, he held a private practice in Portland, Oregon, for twenty-three years with a primary focus on the management of chronic disease, including autoimmune disease, neurological conditions, gastrointestinal problems, and endocrine disorders. For the last five years he has focused on building a state-of-the-art clinic for biological medicine in Scottsdale, Arizona. The American Center for Biological Medicine now provides exceptional care to all patients from young babies to the elderly.

Dr. James Paul Maffitt Odell, OMD, ND, L.Ac., began his medical career as a hospital respiratory therapist while in undergraduate studies in biology at Texas Tech University. Disillusioned with conventional medicine, he focused his attention on natural medicine and graduated from Alliant International University with a doctorate in naturopathy in 1980, after which he studied traditional Chinese medicine and Mandarin Chinese. Having gained conversational fluency in Mandarin, he moved to China in 1986, where he completed a three-year postdoctoral program in traditional Chinese medicine at Shantou University Medical College, with medical residencies at Shantou University Teaching Hospital, Shantou Central Hospital, and Shiwan Hospital. Upon returning from China, he completed several internships in European biological regulatory medicine at the Paracelsus Klinik in Lustmühle, Switzerland.

Dr. Odell is certified in acupuncture with the National Certification Commission for Acupuncture and Oriental Medicine (NCCAOM) and is a professional development activity provider with the NCCAOM. He is licensed in acupuncture in Kentucky, Colorado, South Carolina, and Utah. For over twenty-five years he has been a certified instructor with the American Organization of Bodywork Therapies of Asia. He is also a certified traditional naturopath with the American Naturopathic Certification Board.

For over fifteen years Dr. Odell was the education coordinator for the Bioregulatory Medicine Network, and helped to conduct conferences on the principles and practices of European biological regulatory medicine. He is currently the medical director of the Bioregulatory Medicine Institute. He is also a medical consultant for PDC Biological Health Group and conducts workshops on contact regulation thermography interpretation. In addition to having a busy health care practice, Dr. Odell is the owner and CEO of Phytodyne of Kentucky Inc., which is the North American importer and distributor of Ceres Heilmittel AG plant remedies manufactured in Switzerland.

Dr. Jeoffery Drobot, NMD, is one of the cofounders and medical directors at the American Center for Biological Medicine

(ACBM) in Scottsdale, Arizona. Dr. Drobot also sees patients at his Canadian clinic in Calgary, Alberta, where he has practiced for sixteen years. He graduated from the University of Calgary with a degree in exercise physiology in 1997 and then received a doctorate degree from the National University of Naturopathic Medicine in Portland, Oregon, graduating in 2001. He has spent the last twenty years learning from the best and seeking out cutting-edge science and technology to assess and amplify human biology and physiology. Dr. Drobot works closely with amateur and professional athletes as well as organizations and companies interested in peak performance and longevity.

A leading authority in the field of bioregulatory medicine, Dr. Drobot has decades of experiencing working with chronic and autoimmune disease treatments, detoxification, hormonal imbalance correction, and customized sports medicine and nutrition programs. His love of medicine has evolved into a vast clinical focus treating men, women, and children from the youngest to the oldest. A passion for learning has regularly led him to travel the world attending seminars, educating others, and spending time with the most talented people in medicine. He has partnerships with the exclusive resort community Albany, in the Bahamas, Made Foods in Calgary, as well as various other health and wellness organizations around the world. When not traveling the globe on one of his multiple health ventures or with professional sports teams, Dr. Drobot can also be found at www.drdrobot.com, where he has an active, live Q&A and educational video portal focusing on high-level health education and guidance.

Dr. Frank Pleus, MD, DDS, OMFS, is a Swiss physician and has earned degrees in dentistry and medicine. His training in integrative medicine took place in Switzerland, followed by dental education in Germany and Switzerland; medical education in Germany, Sweden, and Switzerland; and oral and maxillofacial surgery training in Germany and Switzerland. As part of his education, Dr. Pleus trained as a general practitioner in internal and family medicine, gastroenterology, medical psychology, neuraltherapy, orthomolecular medicine, phytotherapy, and naturopathic treatments. He is the author of many doctoral papers on dentistry and medicine.

Dr. Pleus has been one of the key academic lecturers on bioregulatory medicine for the Bioregulatory Medicine Network at the Marion Institute in Marion, Massachusetts. For more than a decade, he has introduced the core precepts and practices of bioregulatory medicine at the annual spring meetings of the network. Doctors, dentists, naturopaths, and lay attendees have learned about bioregulatory medicine and its healing methodologies, as well as approaches in personalized medical practice that can further restore the body and prevent illness.

Dr. Pleus's very unique medical practice, Concièrge Medical Services Switzerland, offers personalized integrative medicine and dentistry, health case management, prevention, and rehabilitation. Dr. Pleus's concept emphasizes truly spending time with patients, listening to their histories, and looking at interactions among various genetic, environmental, and lifestyle factors that can influence long-term health, heal chronic-multiplex diseases, and create awareness for preventive behavior. As a European integrative medicine practitioner, Dr. Pleus firmly believes that maintaining health and healing means integrating all levels of human existence.

Jess Higgins Kelley, MNT, is the founder and CEO of Remission Nutrition, a global oncology nutrition consulting and education enterprise. In addition to pioneering the field of oncology nutrition, Kelley—an oncology nutrition consultant—has been instrumental in the development of various nationally certified nutrition education programs for both the general public and practitioners. With an undergraduate degree in journalism, Kelley has written health and nutrition articles for a multitude of local and national publications and is also the coauthor of *The Metabolic Approach to Cancer* (Chelsea Green, 2017).